Hospital Images

Hospital Images
A Clinical Atlas

Edited by

Paul B. Aronowitz, MD, FACP
Department of Medicine, California Pacific Medical Center, San Francisco

WILEY-BLACKWELL

A John Wiley & Sons, Inc., Publication

Published by John Wiley & Sons, Inc., Hoboken, New Jersey.
Published simultaneously in Canada.

For general information on our other products and services or for technical support, please contact our
Customer Care Department within the United States at (800) 762-2974, outside the United States at
(317) 572-3993 or fax (317) 572-4002.

Wiley also publishes its books in a variety of electronic formats. Some content that appears in print
may not be available in electronic formats. For more information about Wiley products, visit our web
site at www.wiley.com.

Library of Congress Cataloging-in-Publication Data:
Aronowitz, Paul.
   Hospital images : a clinical atlas / Paul Aronowitz.
      p. ; cm.
   Includes bibliographical references.
   ISBN 978-0-470-50101-6 (pbk.)
1. Diagnostic imaging–Atlases.   2. Diagnostic imaging–Examinations, questions, etc.   3. Diagnostic
imaging–Case studies.   I. Title.
   [DNLM: 1. Diagnosis–Atlases.   2. Diagnosis–Case Reports.   3. Emergency
Medicine.   4. Patient Care Management.   WB 17]
   RC78.7.D53A763 2011
   616.07'5–dc23

                                                                2011021005

Printed in Singapore.

10 9 8 7 6 5 4 3 2 1

To Cam, Anna, and Brian with all my love

At the White Window

Whatever one sees beyond it—
green lawn, gray sky, blue heaving sea—

it's clear that the window's framing of the view
is half the meaning, maybe more.

The room is bare, the floorboards simple,
the sunlight falls in angles on the floor.

By being here alone, our sight
entering this picture, thoughtfully,

we celebrate both solitude and its mysterious
opposite, the sense of never being quite alone,

of having dim companions—from the past,
the future, from unsensed dimensions—

as we move slowly to the window,
never to raise the sash, or even touch the pane,

but simply to look out, acknowledging
our unabashed humanity, both frame and view.

—David Young, from *At the White Window*
(Ohio State University Press, 2000)

Contents

Preface

The clinical images and the questions that accompany this book's images are presented in no particular order. They are presented in the same way that patients present to health-care teams taking care of them in the hospital—randomly. During rounds, a hospitalist moves from one patient with a unique set of problems and illnesses to the next patient with a completely different set of unique issues and illnesses. One patient may have a clinical finding easily diagnosed and treated while another may have a complex finding that baffles the hospitalist and the rest of the team for days or even weeks. Learning in medicine is mostly random. I believe that we learn best when fed information in small bite-size pieces that we can reflect on and absorb and when these pieces of learning are directly tied to the patients we or our colleagues are caring for. I have tried to adhere to this principle in creating this book. The questions are meant to challenge the reader and the answers are intended to teach or reinforce a few small pieces of related information. I hope that you, the reader, learn a few things from this book and, most important, I hope you are able to take better care of your patients somewhere down the road because that which you learned was helpful.

This book would not have been possible without the help and support of the residents and chief residents who have trained at California Pacific Medical Center in San Francisco. I would also be remiss if I didn't thank the attending physicians who have been such excellent colleagues and doctors over the last 16 years at California Pacific Medical Center. Finally, I wish to acknowledge and to thank our patients. I hope that the reader learns a few things from this book and I hope that these bits of knowledge will help the reader to take better care of patients in the future since that's what it's all about.

Note: Any royalties generated by sales of this book will be divided between two nonprofit organizations, the Association of Program Directors of Internal Medicine (APDIM) and Oberlin College.

APDIM is the preeminent organization dedicated to the education and training of internal medicine residents and to supporting program directors and program administrators as they strive to mold excellent physicians in a rapidly evolving health-care environment. Without APDIM and the terrific friends and colleagues from APDIM I have met and collaborated with over the years, I could never have done my job or been a program director this long—a decade.

Oberlin College, located in the great state of Ohio, was an important stop on the "Underground Railroad" and was one of the first liberal arts colleges in the United States to admit and degree African Americans and women.

P. B. Aronowitz

Case 1

Image contributed by Sara Thierman

A 38-year-old woman who is 14 months postpartum and still nursing her baby presents to the Emergency Department with 1 day of right breast pain, erythema, and fever consistent with mastitis. She reports that she was told she had a rash when given penicillin as a child and has avoided penicillin and penicillin-related antibiotics since then. She is admitted to one of your colleagues on the hospitalist service and begun on vancomycin and ceftriaxone. Twenty-four hours later, while you are working on the "nocturnist" shift, you are contacted by her nurse and asked to assess this patient for a new rash. She has numerous nonfollicular pustules around her mouth and on her chin, posterior neck (Fig. 1.1), and upper back; she describes them as itchy and burning.

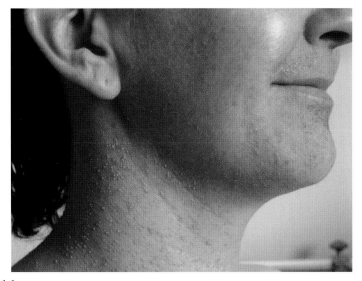

Figure 1.1

Hospital Images: A Clinical Atlas, First Edition. Edited by Paul B. Aronowitz.
© 2012 Wiley-Blackwell. Published 2012 by John Wiley & Sons, Inc.

Question

This patient has which of the following conditions:

- **A.** Pustular psoriasis
- **B.** Drug hypersensitivity syndrome (also known as drug rash with eosinophilia and systemic symptoms [DRESS])
- **C.** Toxic epidermal necrolysis (TEN)
- **D.** Acute generalized exanthematous pustulosis (AGEP)

Answer: D

This patient has AGEP, a rare skin eruption caused by medications in 90% of cases. It is characterized by the acute eruption of many nonfollicular, pustular lesions over erythrodermic skin. The majority of reported cases occur in the setting of aminopenicillin or macrolide antibiotic use, but occasionally AGEP has been caused by drugs such as hydroxychloroquine, carbamazepine, calcium channel blockers, and herbal medicines. Sulfonamides have not been associated with this disorder. Less than 10% of cases have been attributed to viral infections, dietary supplements, and hypersensitivity reactions to spider bites and mercury and radiation exposure.

Acute generalized exanthematous pustulosis can occur 1–3 weeks after administration of a new drug but also, as with this patient previously sensitized to penicillin, in as little as hours to 2–3 days later. Culture of pustules is sterile and skin biopsy reveals spongiform subcorneal and intraepidermal pustules as well as perivascular infiltration with neutrophils and eosinophils. Treatment is cessation of the offending drug and consideration of intravenous or oral steroids. Since the course of this disorder is quite benign after the drug is stopped, some authors recommend avoiding steroid therapy. The pustular lesions usually resolve after 1–3 weeks.

Although this rash may potentially be confused with pustular psoriasis, the acute onset and association with antibiotic administration make AGEP far more likely. Drug hypersensitivity syndrome, also known as drug rash with eosinophilia and systemic symptoms (DRESS), can present with pustular lesions but also occurs with peripheral eosinophilia, lymphadenopathy, fever, mononucleosis-like symptoms, and other visceral involvement such as hepatitis and pneumonitis. TEN can sometimes be confused with this disorder, but AGEP tends to be more superficial with less skin sloughing. Mucous membrane involvement can occur in AGEP but tends to be much less severe than with TEN; pathology usually helps to distinguish the two—TEN typically showing full-thickness epidermal necrolysis.

In this case, ceftriaxone was immediately discontinued, and the patient was switched to clindamycin and started on a corticosteroid taper. Her lesions resolved over the next several days.

Choi MJ, et al. Clinicopathologic manifestations of 36 Korean patients with acute generalized exanthematous pustulosis: a case series and review of the literature. *Ann Dermatol* 2010;22(2):163–169.
Sidoroff A, et al. Acute generalized exanthematous pustulosis (AGEP)—a clinical reaction pattern. *J Cutan Pathol* 2001;28:113–119.

Case 2

A 73-year-old woman with a history of advanced breast cancer metastatic to lung and bone is transferred to your team in the Intensive Care Unit (ICU) from the Medical ward, for bronchospasm and respiratory distress. In the ICU, she receives oxygen, furosemide, and nebulized bronchodilators through a face mask connected to a noninvasive positive pressure ventilator (NIPPV). On the second day of her ICU stay you are contacted by her nurse and informed that your patient's right pupil is fixed and dilated at 4 mm (Fig. 2.1). You perform a careful physical examination and find that she does not have any other focal neurologic abnormalities but that she is sleepy and has diffuse wheezes and rales.

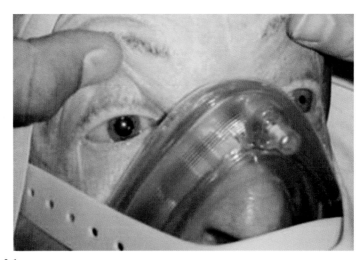

Figure 2.1

Hospital Images: A Clinical Atlas, First Edition. Edited by Paul B. Aronowitz.
© 2012 Wiley-Blackwell. Published 2012 by John Wiley & Sons, Inc.

Question

What is the best subsequent step in this patient's management?

A. Obtain a stat computed tomographic (CT) scan of the brain to rule out acute cerebral hemorrhage.

B. Obtain stat magnetic resonance imaging (MRI) of the brain to look for metastatic brain lesions with uncal herniation.

C. Stop nebulized bronchodilator therapy and observe.

D. Assume this patient has physiologic anisocoria, which is present in 19% of people; continue all current therapy; and intubate the patient for declining respiratory status.

Answer: C

Although this patient is certainly at risk of metastatic spread of her breast cancer to her brain, your careful neurologic examination helps to exclude a central cause for her anisocoria and narrow the etiology to a peripheral cause. Though combined therapy with aerosolized β-2-agonists and anticholinergic agents to treat bronchospasm is still somewhat controversial, combination use is increasingly common in the acute-care setting. Improperly fitting face masks or improper aim of handheld nebulizers can expose the eyes to these medications. Ipratroprium bromide is a derivative of atropine that directly antagonizes muscarinic cholinergic receptors. Inadvertent administration to the eye paralyzes the parasympathetic nerve endings and results in mydriasis. If this patient was not somnolent from her declining respiratory status, she probably would have complained of unilateral blurring of her vision. Bronchodilators were discontinued and this patient's mydriasis resolved by the following day. She was subsequently changed to comfort care and died peacefully.

Dilation of a single pupil can be caused by a mydriatic drug, cranial nerve 3 paralysis, or increased intraocular pressure from acute glaucoma. Although around 19% of the healthy population has physiologic anisocoria at baseline, a fixed, mydriatic pupil narrows the differential diagnosis considerably. Dilation and constriction of the affected pupil would still occur with physiologic anisicoria.

LAM BL, THOMPSON HS, CORBETT JJ. The prevalence of of simple anisocoria. *Am J Ophthalmol* 1987;104(1):69–73.

LOSSON N. Nebulizer-associated anisocoria. *N Engl J Med* 2006;354(9):e8.

LUST K, LIVINGSTONE I. Nebulizer-induced anisocoria. *Ann Intern Med* 1998;128(4):327.

Case 3

Image contributed by Vanessa Gastwirth

A 53-year-old man is admitted to your service for advanced liver failure secondary to chronic active hepatitis B infection. The fourth-year medical student subintern on your team finishes assessing the patient and asks you whether the patient should undergo an evaluation for Addison disease, given his abnormal skin pigmentation (Fig. 3.1).

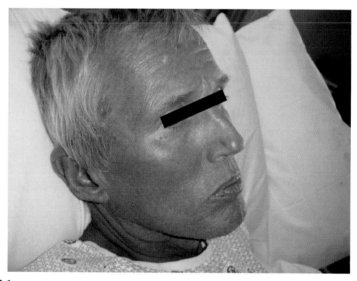

Figure 3.1

Hospital Images: A Clinical Atlas, First Edition. Edited by Paul B. Aronowitz.
© 2012 Wiley-Blackwell. Published 2012 by John Wiley & Sons, Inc.

Question

After obtaining additional medical history and examining the patient, which of the following would you expect this patient to tell you?

A. He has had abdominal pain, weakness, and fatigue.

B. His primary care physician expressed concern that he has concurrent Wilson disease and chronic active hepatitis B infection.

C. He has chronic hypoxemia from a long history of tobacco use.

D. He has been chronically ingesting a "cure-all" that contains silver colloid, sold over the Internet.

Answer: D

This patient's skin examination is remarkable for generalized argyria. The term "argyria" comes from the Greek word for silver. Further history revealed that he had learned to produce a silver colloid solution using a car battery and silver electrical wire purchased from an Internet site.

The medicinal use of silver dates back to the eighth century and the term argyria was probably first used in 1840 by Fuchs. Prior to the development of antibiotics, silver was frequently used to treat colds, sinusitis, mental illness, epilepsy, nicotine addiction, eye irritation, and infectious diseases, including syphilis and gonorrhea. Due to its antibacterial effects, it is still used in silver sulfadiazine cream to treat burns; however, the use of colloidal silver and silver salts in over-the-counter medications was banned by the US Food and Drug Administration (FDA) in 1999. Extremely large doses of silver can cause central nervous system toxicity, but there is little definitive evidence that the deposition of silver in vital organs causes anything other than cosmetic harm.

Generalized argyria is almost always caused by ingestion of soluble silver compounds. As it is deposited in the skin, light converts it to silver salts that cause an irreversible silver or blue-grey color. This pigmentation is especially pronounced in sun-exposed areas of the body.

Pigmentation may also occur in the eyes, which is known as argyrosis. Localized argyria has been described as a consequence of the use of acupuncture needles, silver earrings, catheters, and dental amalgams.

Although Addison disease might be in the differential diagnosis, primary adrenal insufficiency causes browning or darkening of skin, particularly in the creases of hands, extensor surfaces, nipples, and buccal mucosa. Other etiologies to consider in the differential diagnosis include Wilson disease, methemoglobinemia, carcinoid syndrome, hemochromatosis, and ingestion of compounds or metals such as antimalarials, amiodarone, tetracyclines, gold, mercury, and bismuth.

DRAKE PL, HAZELWOOD KJ. Exposure-related health effects of silver and silver compounds: a review. *Ann Occupational Hyg* 2005;49(7):575–585.
WADHERA A, FUNG M. Systemic argyria associated with ingestion of colloidal silver. *Dermatol Online J* 2005;11(1):12–22.

Case 4

Image contributed by Albert Lu

A 67-year-old woman is admitted to the hospital for hematemesis and melena. Her blood pressure is 80/70 mmHg and pulse is 112 beats per minute, and she complains of dizziness when standing. Nasogastric lavage reveals a small amount of "coffee ground" material that clears after 500 cc of saline lavage. Her hematocrit is 31%; 1 month prior to admission it was 38%, seen during a routine visit to her primary care physician.

Her admission chest radiograph does not reveal any acute disease (Fig. 4.1). She is admitted to the medical Intensive Care Unit (ICU) and is given intravenous fluid resuscitation and proton pump inhibitor medication. A gastroenterology consultant performs an upper endoscopy after administering 2 mg of midazolam and 50 mg of meperidine for conscious sedation. Endoscopic examination reveals a duodenal ulcer with a clean base and no active bleeding. The procedure is completed without apparent complications. Approximately 30 minutes after the procedure, an ICU nurse contacts you because the patient's oxygen saturation is 84% and her

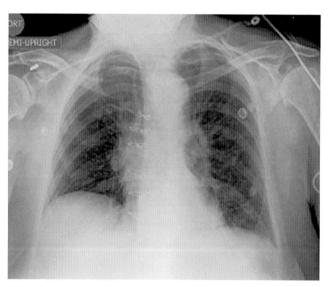

Figure 4.1   Admission chest radiograph.

Hospital Images: A Clinical Atlas, First Edition. Edited by Paul B. Aronowitz.
© 2012 Wiley-Blackwell. Published 2012 by John Wiley & Sons, Inc.

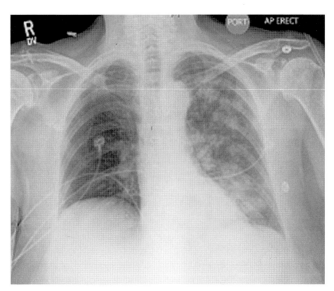

Figure 4.2   Postprocedure chest radiograph.

respiratory rate is 32 breaths per minute. Her blood pressure is 144/88 mmHg. As you arrive to evaluate the patient, the nurse notes that she has a fever of 38.9°C. A repeat chest radiograph is obtained (Fig. 4.2).

Question 1

Which of the following is the best subsequent step in the management of this patient?

A. Order broad-spectrum intravenous antibiotics that cover anaerobic, aerobic, and gram-negative bacterial pathogens.

B. Order oxygen, continue proton pump inhibitors, and observe.

C. Order oxygen, broad-spectrum antibiotics, and a dysphagia evaluation by speech therapy.

D. Intubate the patient and administer 100% O_2 via endotracheal tube.

Question 2

Choose the statement that best defines the difference between aspiration pneumonia and aspiration pneumonitis:

A. They are essentially the same thing with major areas of overlap; differentiating these entities has little or no clinical significance.

B. Aspiration pneumonitis involves the aspiration of oral contents containing bacteria into the lungs, always resulting in aspiration pneumonia 2–7 days later.

C. Due to advanced anesthetic techniques, aspiration pneumonitis is no longer a cause of death from general anesthesia.

D. Aspiration pneumonitis is a chemical injury caused by the inhalation of sterile gastric contents; aspiration pneumonia is an infectious process caused by the inhalation of oropharyngeal secretions that are colonized by pathogenic bacteria.

Answer 1: B

This patient has aspiration pneumonitis, which likely occurred due to conscious sedation and her procedure. Aspiration in adults is usually due to loss of protective reflexes in the setting of altered consciousness or impaired neuromuscular function. Aspiration pneumonitis is a noninfectious inflammatory response due to the aspiration of sterile gastric contents, which does not usually require antimicrobial treatment. It can cause anything from mild to severe respiratory impairment. Initial management includes careful monitoring for at least 12 hours after the aspiration event. Antibiotics should be considered if the patient develops purulent sputum, fever persisting beyond the initial aspiration event, or other signs and symptoms of pneumonia.

Answer 2: D

Aspiration pneumonitis results from aspiration of sterile, acidic gastric contents, whereas aspiration pneumonia occurs due to the aspiration of oral secretions that are colonized by potentially pathogenic bacteria. The aspiration of oral contents into the lungs does not always result in pneumonia. However, patients who have aspirated gastric contents may present with shortness of breath, fever, hypoxemia, pulmonary edema, hypotension, cough, and wheezing and occasionally progress to respiratory failure from adult respiratory distress syndrome.

Aspiration pneumonitis, or Mendelson's syndrome, was reported in 1946 in patients who developed aspiration pneumonitis after general anesthesia during obstetrical procedures. Aspiration pneumonitis can be a complication of general anesthesia and occurs in approximately 1 in 3000 operations where anesthesia is administered. Aspiration pneumonitis accounts for 10–30% of all deaths associated with anesthesia.

MARIK PE. Aspiration pneumonitis and aspiration pneumonia. *N Engl J Med* 2001;344(9):665–671.
PAINTAL HS, KUSCHNER WG. Aspiration syndromes: 10 clinical pearls every physician should know. *Int J Clin Pract* 2007;61(5):846–852.

Case 5

Image contributed by Emmanuel King

A 75-year-old male from rural southern New Jersey was admitted for fever of unknown origin. On hospital day 2 his hemoglobin dropped from 11.3 g/dL to 7.5 g/dL, with an associated elevated indirect bilirubin and lactate dehydrogenase. He also developed hypoxia and lethargy. A blood smear showed numerous intracellular and extracellular abnormalities, with approximately 30% of his red blood cells involved (Fig. 5.1).

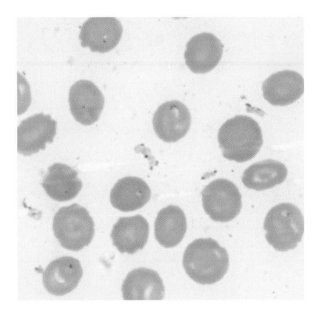

Figure 5.1

Hospital Images: A Clinical Atlas, First Edition. Edited by Paul B. Aronowitz.
© 2012 Wiley-Blackwell. Published 2012 by John Wiley & Sons, Inc.

Question 1

Which of the following is the most appropriate subsequent step in this patient's management?

A. Intravenous ceftriaxone

B. Intravenous doxycycline

C. Emergent dialysis

D. Intravenous clindamycin, quinine, and red blood cell exchange transfusion

The patient's daughter is concerned because she and her 8-year-old son have been spending much of the summer with the patient at his rural home, and she wants to know if she and her son should see their family doctor or take antibiotics.

Question 2

What would be your next step or advice to the patient's daughter?

A. Prescribe the patient's daughter and her son a 7-day course of doxycycline.

B. Contact the New Jersey Department of Public Health to report the patient's illness and seek further advice concerning his daughter and grandson.

C. Reassure the patient's daughter, educate her about methods of preventing exposure to this disease, and advise her to see a physician for flulike symptoms.

D. Administer a single 250-mg dose of intramuscular ceftriaxone.

Answer 1: D

This patient is severely ill with babesiosis, an emerging tick-borne disease caused by the protozoa *Babesia*. *Babesia* species belong to the phylum Apicomplexa, which also includes *Plasmodium* species, which cause malaria. There are over 100 species of *Babesia*, with two species causing most human infections—*B. microti* and *B. divergens*. *Babesia microti* is the main species encountered in the United States. The white-footed mouse (*Peromyscus leucopus*) is the principal reservoir for *B. microti*, and in some endemic areas two-thirds of white-footed mice are parasitemic. The disease is transmitted from mouse to human by the tick *Ixodes scapularis*, which can also transmit Lyme disease. Endemic areas include coastal areas and islands of Massachusetts and New York as well as areas of Connecticut and New Jersey. The *Ixodes* tick also feeds on white-tailed deer, though the deer are not a reservoir for *Babesia*. The population boom in deer, an important food source for *Ixodes* ticks, is thought to be playing a role in the emergence and growing prevalence of babesiosis in the Northeast. This disease is also emerging in areas of Connecticut, California, and Washington. Of note, one-fourth of patients with babesiosis are also infected with *Borrelia burgdorferi*, the causative agent of Lyme disease also carried by *I. scapularis* ticks.

Most cases of babesiosis occur in the spring and summer and the incubation period is from 1 to 4 weeks. Infection with *Babesia microti* is usually asymptomatic. However, elderly, asplenic, and immunosuppressed patients are most at risk of systemic illness. Flulike symptoms, including fever, headache, myalgias, and malaise, may occur for weeks and even up to months. Hepatosplenomegaly, jaundice, and dark urine may be present on physical examination, and thrombocytopenia, leukopenia, and hemolytic anemia may be present on laboratory testing. Acute respiratory distress syndrome is sometimes seen in severe cases.

This patient was quite ill at the time of presentation and was treated with intravenous antibiotics and red blood cell exchange transfusion. Treatment options include clindamycin with quinine or atovaquone with azithromycin—the latter regimen having a better side-effect profile. This patient's clinical status markedly improved and he was subsequently discharged home.

Babesiosis should be considered in the differential diagnosis of hemolytic anemia in patients that live in or have traveled to endemic areas. The most common appearance on blood smear is round to oval rings with pale blue cytoplasm and a red-staining nucleus. Pathognomonic "Maltese cross" tetrad forms (uncommon) or extra-erythrocytic parasites as well as a detailed travel history help to differentiate babesiosis from malaria.

Answer 2: C

Most patients infected with this disease are asymptomatic. A concerned patient or family member should be reassured and educated about avoiding tick bites and doing "tick checks" after outdoor activities, and about rashes and symptoms that could be due to either babesiosis or Lyme disease. Babesiosis is not a reportable disease. Prophylactic antibiotics are not recommended for babesiosis. It is unlikely that ceftriaxone or doxycycline alone would be adequate to treat or prevent babesiosis.

BLEVINS SM, GREEENFIELD RA, BRONZE MS. Blood smear analysis in babesiosis, ehrlichiosis, relapsing fever, malaria and Chagas disease. *Clev Clin J Med* 2008;75(7);521–530.

KING E, et al. Severe babesiosis. *J Hosp Med* 2010;5(5):E8.

VANNIER E, GEWURZ BE, KRAUSE PJ. Human babesiosis. *Infect Dis Clin North Am* 2008;22:469–488.

Case 6

Image contributed by Sara Thierman

You are called for a medical consultation by a cardiologist. His patient is a 57-year-old woman who developed a pruritic rash 6 hours after undergoing coronary angiography. She had a previous angiography 1 year ago, after she presented with an ST-segment elevation myocardial infarction. She had been having atypical chest pain in recent weeks and was admitted to the hospital to rule out another myocardial infarction. Her current medications include aspirin and metoprolol, which she has been taking for several years. On physical examination, the patient is anxious about her rash but in no distress. Symmetrical erythematous plaques are noted in bilateral inguinal areas (Fig. 6.1), buttocks, axillae (Fig. 6.2), and the intertriginous folds of her breasts. Laboratory studies are normal.

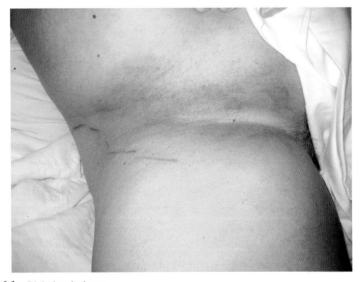

Figure 6.1   Right inguinal area.

Hospital Images: A Clinical Atlas, First Edition. Edited by Paul B. Aronowitz.
© 2012 Wiley-Blackwell. Published 2012 by John Wiley & Sons, Inc.

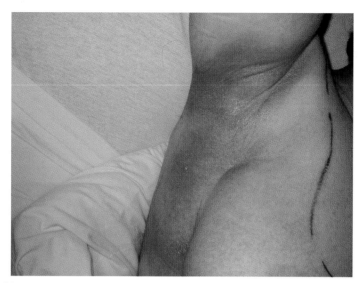

Figure 6.2   Right axilla.

Question

What would you recommend to the cardiologist caring for this patient?

    A. Administer diphenhydramine and avoid iodine-based contrast studies in the future.

    B. Administer diphenhydramine and epinephrine 1:1000 subcutaneously to prevent anaphylaxis.

    C. Stop metoprolol.

    D. Stop aspirin and switch to clopidogrel.

Answer: A

This woman has symmetrical drug-related intertriginous and flexural exanthema (SDRIFE) secondary to iodine-based contrast dye received during her coronary angiogram. This is a type IV hypersensitivity reaction that has been described with numerous drugs, including β-lactam antibiotics (most common), allopurinol, nonsteroidal anti-inflammatory drugs, heparin, topical medications, systemic steroids, and various other medications. This patient had likely been sensitized to iodine 1 year previously, but in many cases previous sensitization is not identified. Previously known as baboon syndrome because its distribution resembles the pink bottom of a baboon, SDRIFE may appear hours to days after exposure to an offending drug or agent. The symmetric and unusual distribution of this rash is probably explained by high concentrations of the offending agent in sweat. This is not a life-threatening disorder and conservative management with antihistamines and "tincture of time" will result in resolution. Oral corticosteroids are sometimes used in more severe reactions. It would be best to avoid the use of iodine-based contrast in this patient in the future.

DHINGRA B, GROVER C. Baboon syndrome. *Ind Pediat* 2007;44:937.

THIERMAN S, CHINTHRAJAH RS. Symmetrical drug-related intertriginous and flexural exanthema after coronary artery angiography. *J Hosp Med* 2009;4(3):203.

TREUDLER R, SIMON JC. Symmetric, drug-related, intertriginous, and flexural exanthema in a patient with polyvalent intolerance to corticosteroids. *J Allergy Clin Immunol* 2006;188(4):965–967.

Case 7

A 70-year-old woman who has a long history of tobacco use is admitted from her primary care physician's office for complaints of progressively worsening headache over several weeks and an outpatient computed tomographic (CT) scan of the head showing a right, cortical, 4.8-cm mass with midline shift (Fig. 7.1, long arrow) and adjacent hemorrhage (Fig. 7.1, short arrow). Magnetic resonance imaging (MRI) with gadolinium enhancement (Fig. 7.2) is done shortly after admission and it does not show any other lesions.

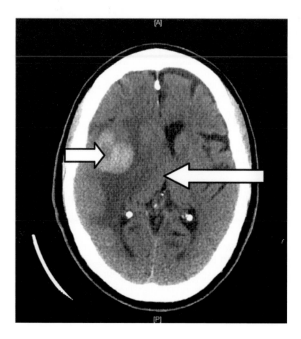

Figure 7.1

Hospital Images: A Clinical Atlas, First Edition. Edited by Paul B. Aronowitz.
© 2012 Wiley-Blackwell. Published 2012 by John Wiley & Sons, Inc.

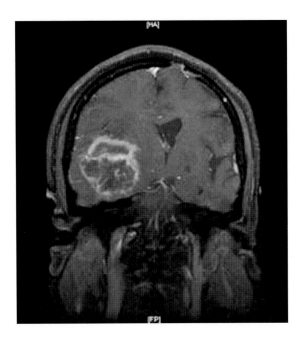

Figure 7.2

Question 1

The patient asks you whether you think she has primary brain cancer. Prior to obtaining other tests, what would you tell her?

    A. She most likely has a primary brain tumor.

    B. She is more likely to have metastatic disease to the brain from a systemic cancer.

    C. There is about a 50–50 chance that the brain tumor could be primary brain cancer or metastatic disease.

A chest radiograph reveals a left lung 17 × 9-cm mass (Fig. 7.3, arrow) and right hilar prominence. A CT-guided fine needle aspiration of the left lung mass reveals non-small-cell lung carcinoma (NSCLC), and the CT scan reveals two nodules in the right middle lobe consistent with metastatic disease and enlarged hilar lymph nodes.

Question 2

Other than reviewing this patient's advance care directive, which of the following would be the best subsequent step in this patient's care?

    A. Begin dexamethasone and consult Radiation–Oncology for whole-brain radiation.

    B. Begin dexamethasone and antiseizure medication, and consult Oncology and Neurosurgery to discuss chemotherapy with possible surgical resection of the brain mass.

    C. Begin antiseizure medication and perform a lumbar puncture, checking opening pressure and sending cerebrospinal fluid for cell count and cytology.

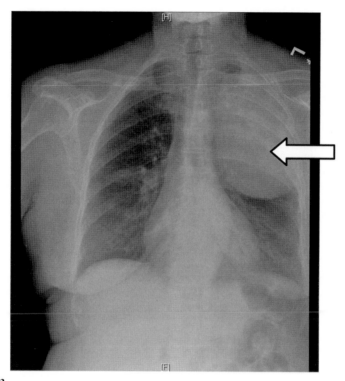

Figure 7.3

    D. Initiate palliative care and treat the patient with whatever analgesics and antiemetics
are required to keep her comfortable.

Question 3

In patients with brain metastases, which of the following is the most important *favorable*
prognostic factor?

    A. Type of cancer

    B. Having less than three co-morbid conditions

    C. Having a high performance status

    D. Being less than 60 years of age

Answer 1: B

Brain metastases are up to 10 times more common than primary tumors of the brain. Approximately 20–40% of patients with cancer will eventually develop metastatic disease in the brain. Brain metastases are more frequently diagnosed in patients with known malignancies (metachronous presentation). Up to 30% of brain metastases are diagnosed at the same time as a primary tumor diagnosis (synchronous presentation) and, less commonly, before there is evidence of primary disease (precocious presentation). This patient's presentation would be considered a synchronous presentation given the findings on her chest radiograph at the time of admission.

It is very important to perform a gadolinium-enhanced MRI scan to evaluate for other brain lesions, as CT scans can miss metastases. Knowing the extent and number of metastases may have an impact on treatment and prognosis. However, in general, the prognosis for patients presenting with brain metastases is poor. For patients presenting with single brain lesions that can be resected, the median survival is approximately 10–16 months. For patients with multiple brain metastases the prognosis is approximately 3–6 months.

Answer 2: A

Even though this patient's prognosis is poor given the extent of her systemic cancer (large tumor, metastatic disease to the contralateral lung and brain), she has a headache and midline shift that could very well improve with steroids and palliative whole-brain radiation. Although surgical resection and systemic chemotherapy could be considered, there is no solid evidence that antiseizure medications should be started in patients who have not had seizures. In fact, the risks of drug–drug interactions and drug side effects appear to outweigh the benefits of seizure prophylaxis.

Although moving in the direction of palliative care is not unreasonable, the initiation of steroids and consideration of palliative brain irradiation would be a reasonable next step, depending on the patient's wishes.

Answer 3: C

Various studies have identified favorable prognostic factors in patients with brain metastases. Among these, a high performance status as measured by the Karnofsky performance status (KPS) is the most important factor. A maximum KPS is 100 (normal, no complaints, no evidence of disease) with points deducted in increments of 10 for impact of the disease. For example, a KPS of 70 means the patient is able to care for herself but unable to carry on normal activity or to do active work. Other favorable prognostic factors include whether the brain metastases are solitary, the absence of other systemic metastases, a controlled primary tumor, and age less than 60–65 years old.

Eichler AF, Loeffler J. Multidisciplinary management of brain metastases. *The Oncologist* 2007;12:884–898.
Soffietti R, et al. Management of brain metastases. *J Neurol* 2002;249:1357–1369.

Case 8

An 86-year-old woman with a long history of diabetes mellitus and congestive heart failure is brought to the Emergency Department (ED) by her daughter to be evaluated for 5 days of lower extremity blisters. The ED physician asks you to "take a look" at the patient as she is concerned the patient has cellulitis or "something worse." The patient has not started any new medications recently and states that she "feels fine" and that the blisters are painless. She reports that she has chronic lower extremity edema that is currently at baseline. She says she woke up in the morning 5 days ago and that the blisters were present. Physical examination reveals a pleasant, elderly woman in no distress. Her temperature is 36.5°C and her other vital signs are normal. Bullous lesions are present on both feet (Figs. 8.1 and 8.2) and anterior lower legs up the midshin region. Unroofing one small bulla reveals clear, colorless fluid. Other than a baseline grade II/VI mitral regurgitation murmur and scant bibasilar crackles, the patient's cardiac and pulmonary examination does not reveal signs of congestive heart failure.

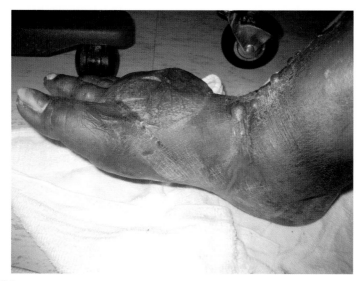

Figure 8.1

Hospital Images: A Clinical Atlas, First Edition. Edited by Paul B. Aronowitz.
© 2012 Wiley-Blackwell. Published 2012 by John Wiley & Sons, Inc.

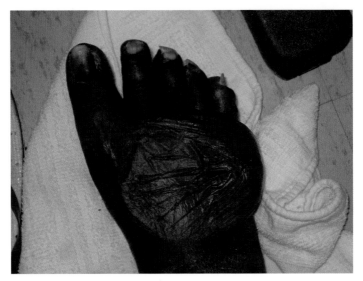

Figure 8.2

The ED is placed on "diversion" status while you are seeing the patient and talking with her daughter. The ED physician thanks you for seeing the patient and asks that you either admit the patient to the hospital or clear her for discharge, as ED beds must cleared of stable patients in order to reverse the ED's diversion status.

Question

What would the best subsequent step be in this patient's management?

    A. Admit her to the hospital for intravenous antibiotics and dermatology consultation.

    B. Admit her to the hospital for intravenous lasix and close monitoring of electrolytes.

    C. Discharge her home with an increased dose of lasix and wound-care instructions.

    D. Discharge her home with wound-care instructions, reassurance, and referral to a dermatologist for consideration of skin biopsy.

Answer: D

This patient has bullosis diabeticorum, a very poorly understood blistering skin condition that occurs in the distal extremities of diabetic patients. These blisters are usually painless but can sometimes cause a burning sensation. They frequently arise overnight and are usually not associated with trauma. Lower extremity edema, peripheral vascular disease, diabetic neuropathy, and kidney disease have all been associated with this disorder. Skin biopsy and electron miroscopic studies reveal that these blisters are usually subepidermal at the level of the lamina lucida. Other diagnoses that should be considered in this patient include a drug reaction, porphyria cutanea tarda, and immunobullous disorders such as epidermolysis bullosa acquisita.

This patient does not need to be admitted to the hospital. She and her daughter should receive wound-care instructions, reassurance, and close follow-up with her primary care physician or a dermatologist. This condition usually resolves spontaneously in 2–4 weeks.

BASARAB T, et al. Bullosis diabeticorum. A case report and literature review. *Clin Exp Derm* 1995;20:218–220.

SIBBALD G, LANDOLT SJ, TOTH D. Chronic complications of diabetes: skin and diabetes. *Endocrin Metab Clin* 1996;25(2):463–472.

Case 9

A 46-year-old woman is admitted by her primary care doctor to your medical ward with complaints of fever of 38.6°C along with redness, swelling, and pain over her left elbow. She is otherwise healthy and works as a public school teacher. Physical examination reveals a pleasant woman appearing her stated age and in no distress. She has erythema and induration over her left elbow (Fig. 9.1) and a palpable, symmetric fluid collection in that same location (Fig. 9.2). Active and passive range of motion testing of her left elbow fail to elicit pain except at complete flexion and complete extension of the arm.

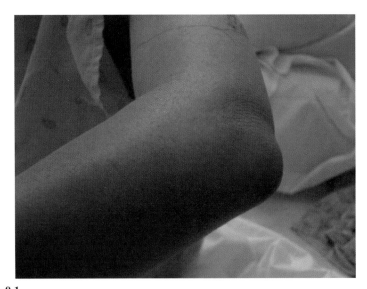

Figure 9.1

Hospital Images: A Clinical Atlas, First Edition. Edited by Paul B. Aronowitz.
© 2012 Wiley-Blackwell. Published 2012 by John Wiley & Sons, Inc.

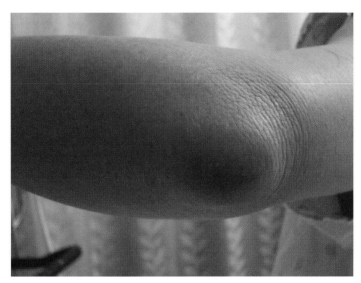

Figure 9.2

Question 1

Which of the following is the most appropriate next step in this patient's management?

    A. Perform left elbow arthrocentesis and send joint fluid for white blood cell count, Gram stain, and culture and start empiric antibiotics.

    B. Begin empiric antibiotics for cellulitis.

    C. Perform needle aspiration of the olecranon bursa and send bursal fluid for white blood cell count, Gram stain, and culture and start empiric antibiotics.

    D. Apply a compression wrap and ice to the left elbow, begin nonsteroidal anti-inflammatory (NSAID) medications, and discharge the patient from the hospital.

Question 2

Regarding the etiology of this disorder, which statement is most accurate?

    A. Approximately 90% of cases are caused by *Staphylococcus aureus*.

    B. Approximately 90% of cases are caused by *Streptococcus pyogenes*.

    C. Approximately 90% of cases are caused by the precipitation of monosodium urate crystals.

    D. Trauma to the elbow is rarely associated with this disorder

Answer 1: C

This patient has septic olecranon bursitis. The appearance of erythema, induration, and swelling over the olecranon process and a fever are consistent with this diagnosis. Although septic arthritis should be considered, lack of pain with passive and active range of motion of the joint in question in an immunocompetent patient makes this diagnosis very unlikely. There is pain elicited at extremes of flexion and extension because the bursa is being stretched in these positions. Cellulitis should also be considered, but swelling of the olecranon bursa makes this less likely. Her occupational history is important since, as a teacher, she likely leans on her elbows a lot, thus causing repetitive trauma to the olecranon bursa (known as student's elbow). Trauma is a frequent precipitating factor. Gardeners, plumbers, custodians, gymnasts, students, and football players are at risk of olecranon bursitis. Septic prepatellar bursitis tends to occur in patients who work on their knees frequently, including coal miners, gardeners, carpet layers, carpenters, and stockers in grocery stores.

The best subsequent step in this patient would be to aspirate the olecranon bursa and send the fluid for white blood cell count, Gram stain, and culture. If the patient is at risk of gout, crystals should also be searched for. Empiric antibiotics should be started pending the results of the Gram stain and cultures. The white blood cell count ranges from >1500 to 418,000 cells per cubic millimeter in septic bursitis but is never less than 1000 cells per cubic millimeter.

Ice, rest, compression dressing, and NSAIDs would be the treatment of choice for non-septic olecranon bursitis. This form of bursitis is usually due to overuse injury or repetitive trauma to the bursa but would not cause fever, as in this patient's case.

Answer 2: A

Staphylococcus aureus is identified in approximately 90% of cases of septic bursitis. *Streptococcus pyogenes* should also be considered but is a less common pathogen. Other unusual pathogens include *Mycobacterium marinum, Sporothrix schenckii, Streptococcus pneumoniae,* and achloric algae. Bursa can also become inflamed without trauma, as with gout. Though gout is a less common etiology of bursitis, fluid should be examined for the presence of crystals in patients at risk of gout.

Most patients with septic olecranon bursitis do well with a 2- to 3-week course of antibiotics and repeat olecranon bursa aspiration as needed to diminish swelling and pain and/or monitor for improvement.

Ho G, et al. Septic bursitis in the prepatellar and olecranon bursae. *Ann Int Med* 1978;89(1):21–27.
SHELL D, PERKINS R, COSGAREA A. Septic olecranon bursitis: recognition and treatment. *J Am Board Fam Pract* 1995;8(3):217–220.

Case 10

Images contributed by Nasim Afsarmanesh

A 38-year-old woman presents to the Emergency Department (ED) with 3 days of drainage from a lesion on her right elbow. An examination of the elbow reveals diffuse and firm subcutaneous nodules with overlying erythema. X-rays illustrate soft-tissue calcifications in the forearm and elbow without evidence of osteomyelitis (Fig. 10.1). Wound cultures subsequently grow *Staphylococcus aureus*, and the patient is started on intravenous antibiotics for treatment.

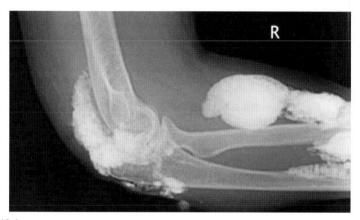

Figure 10.1

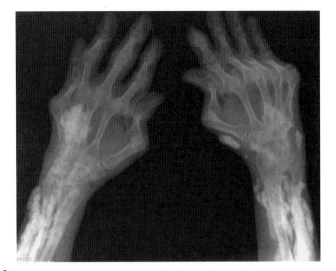

Figure 10.2

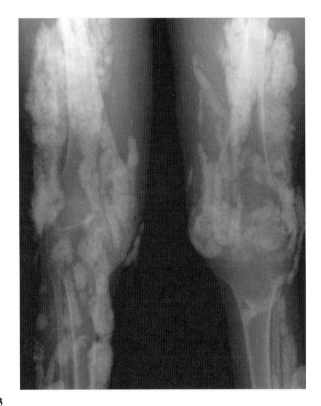

Figure 10.3

Question

This patient's radiographic findings (Figs. 10.1–10.3) are most consistent with which of the following:

A. Calciphylaxis from end-stage kidney disease
B. Hyperparathyroidism
C. Hypercalcemia of malignancy
D. Calcinosis universalis secondary to dermatomyositis

Answer: D

This patient originally presented as a child with juvenile dermatomyositis. Calcinosis universalis is a poorly understood entity associated with various connective tissue disorders, including dermatomyositis, diffuse scleroderma, and Crest syndrome, and it has been described in systemic lupus erythematosus. A common complication of calcinosis universalis is secondary infection by *Staphylococcus aureus* due to skin breakdown. The pathophysiology of this condition is unknown and there is no effective treatment for it.

Calcinosis is classified into four subsets: dystrophic (this case), metastatic, idiopathic, and iatrogenic. In dystrophic calcification, calcium salts are deposited in skin, subcutaneous tissue, muscle, and tendons. Metastatic calcification occurs in tissue when calcium and phosphate levels are elevated (usually when the calcium–phosphate product [serum calcium level multiplied by serum phosphate level] is greater than 70). Calciphylaxis or iatrogenic calcinosis most often occurs in patients on hemodialysis for renal failure.

AFSARMANESH N, GORN A. Calcinosis universalis. *J Hosp Med* 2009;4(1):71–72.
TRISTANO AG, et al. Calcinosis cutis universalis in a patient with systemic lupus erythematosus. *Clin Rheumatol* 2005;25:70–74.

Case 11

Written by Joseph P. Henry

A 46-year-old man with end-stage kidney disease for 5 years who has been on hemodialysis for 5 years is admitted to the vascular surgery service for revision of his arteriovenous fistula. While you are evaluating him as the medical consultant, you note that he has painful nodules on his abdomen and hands (Fig. 11.1). His phosphate is 8.4 mg/dL and his calcium is 10.4 mg/dL. You order a radiograph of the hand (Fig. 11.2).

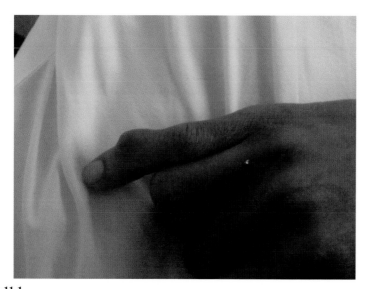

Figure 11.1

Hospital Images: A Clinical Atlas, First Edition. Edited by Paul B. Aronowitz.
© 2012 Wiley-Blackwell. Published 2012 by John Wiley & Sons, Inc.

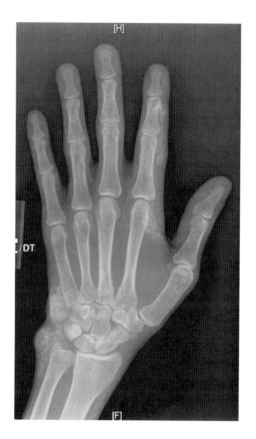

Figure 11.2

Question

What is the most likely diagnosis?

    A. Polyarteritis nodosa

    B. Calciphylaxis

    C. Mixed cryoglobulinemia

    D. Septic emboli from endocarditis

Answer: B

Calciphylaxis is a disorder characterized by systemic calcification of the media in arterioles leading to ischemia and subcutaneous necrosis. It can also cause extravascular calcifications. It is most commonly seen in end-stage kidney disease patients on hemodialysis, but it can also be seen in hyperparathyroidism. Typical clinical manifestations consist of painful necrosis of areas of high adiposity such as the abdomen, buttocks, and thighs as well as digital ischemia. This disorder occurs in approximately 4% of hemodilalysis patients. Calciphylaxis is uncommon in patients with a calcium–phosphate product (serum calcium level multiplied by serum phosphate level) less than 55, but there is not a strong correlation with the exact number as a predictor of this disorder.

ANGELIS M, et al. Calciphylaxis in patients on hemodialysis: a prevalence study. *Surgery* 1997;122(6):1083–1089.

FINE A, ZACHARIAS J. Calciphylaxis is usually non-ulcerating: risk factors, outcome and therapy. *Kid Int* 2002;61(6):2210–2217.

KENT RB, LYERLY RT. Systemic calciphylaxis. *South Med J* 1994;87(2):278–281.

Case 12

Images contributed by Sally Daganzo

A 42-year-old male presents to the Emergency Department several days after developing painful digits of both hands. He denies fevers, chills, sweats, weight loss, and a history of heart murmurs or family diseases, and he has never used intravenous drugs. He has otherwise been in excellent health his entire life. He has smoked 8–10 marijuana cigarettes each day for many years and 1–2 cigarettes per month.

Physical examination reveals a pleasant man complaining of pain in his digits but otherwise well-appearing. He is afebrile, does not have a heart murmur or cutaneous lesions other than those shown in Figure 12.1. He has palpable ulnar and radial pulses and a normal Allen's test. His laboratory studies are normal except for an erythrocyte sedimentation rate of 46, and your resident has ordered and obtained an urgent digital subtraction angiogram (Fig. 12.2) while you were in a long quality-improvement meeting with hospital administrators.

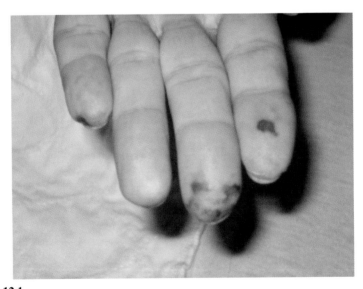

Figure 12.1

Hospital Images: A Clinical Atlas, First Edition. Edited by Paul B. Aronowitz.
© 2012 Wiley-Blackwell. Published 2012 by John Wiley & Sons, Inc.

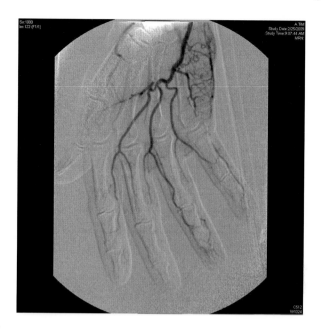

Figure 12.2

Question

Which of the following is the best subsequent step in this patient's management?

    A. Draw blood cultures and initiate intravenous antibiotics, including vancomycin, gentamicin, and ceftriaxone, pending blood culture results.

    B. Order a stat transesophageal echocardiogram and blood cultures.

    C. Administer 1 g of methylprednisolone and begin prednisone 60 mg orally per day.

    D. Counsel the patient that he must immediately discontinue marijuana use or he might eventually need amputation of his digits.

Answer: D

Although this patient's digital macular lesions resemble Janeway lesions seen in endocarditis, his relatively healthy appearance and lack of predisposing risk factors, a fever, or heart murmur make endocarditis a much less likely diagnositic possibility. This patient has cannabis arteritis, a small- and medium-sized artery vasculitis caused by marijuana use that is thought to be a form of thromboangiitis obliterans (Buerger's disease). Cannabis arteritis was first described in 1960 and there are a number of case reports in the medical literature.

The etiology of this vasculitis is unknown, but some authors have highlighted a possible relationship between the presence of arsenic in marijuana and this disorder. In Taiwan, "black-foot disease" is a form of thromboangiitis obliterans that appears to be related to chronic arsenic poisoning from contaminated well water. Arsenic causes dysfunction of endogenous nitric oxide that may then lead to thrombosis and vascular occlusion. Pathologic data about cannabis arteritis are lacking. In thromboangiitis obliterans, all layers of involved vessel walls are initially infiltrated by inflammatory cells, resulting in thrombus formation. Around the periphery of the thrombus, microabscesses may form and giant cells can sometimes be seen.

The course of cannabis arteritis can be quite severe. In at least two case series, 40% of patients with cannabis arteritis required digital amputation. Stopping marijuana is the initial step in treating this disease. Other treatments may include antiplatelet agents, vasodilators such as prostaglandin inhibitors, anticoagulants, hyperbaric oxygen therapy, and occasionally thrombolytics or vascular surgical bypass.

Although initially quite skeptical about the diagnosis, this patient was convinced to permanently discontinue marijuana and his lesions had nearly completely resolved at outpatient follow-up several weeks later.

COMBEMALE P, et al. Cannabis arteritis. *Brit J Dermatol* 2005;152:166–169.

DAGANZO S, NUNE G. Pot shots—cannabis arteritis of the digits. *J Hosp Med* 2010;5(7):424.

NOEL B, RUF I, PANIZZON RG. Cannabis arteritis. *J Am Acad Dermatol* 2008;58:S65–S67.

Case 13

Images contributed by Ernie Lo

A 68-year-old man with a history of hypertension, hyperlipidemia, and peripheral vascular disease is brought to the Emergency Department by ambulance 7 hours after suddenly developing left upper and left lower extremity weakness. Initial neurologic examination reveals a right gaze preference, left-sided neglect, and complete hemiplegia of the left upper and left lower extremities. A computed tomographic (CT) scan (Fig. 13.1) is unrevealing. Because the patient has presented 7 hours after his stroke, the patient is not administered thrombolytic therapy. The patient is admitted to your service in the Intensive Care Unit (ICU), where he is managed with aspirin, a statin medication, and "permissive hypertension."

He is transferred to the medical floors 48 hours after admission, where he is stable with continued dense, left hemiplegia and left neglect. Four days after admission you are contacted by nursing staff because the patient has become increasingly

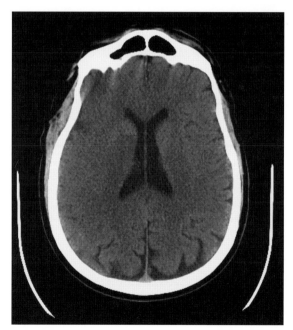

Figure 13.1   Admission CT scan.

Hospital Images: A Clinical Atlas, First Edition. Edited by Paul B. Aronowitz.
© 2012 Wiley-Blackwell. Published 2012 by John Wiley & Sons, Inc.

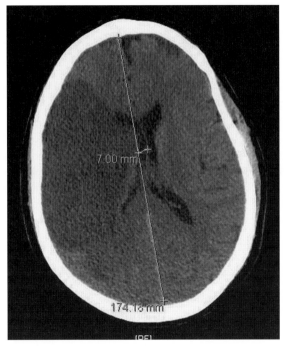

Figure 13.2 CT scan 4 days after admission.

lethargic and difficult to arouse. A head CT scan is done (Fig. 13.2), and the patient is transferred back to the ICU for further management. Shortly after transfer to the ICU he becomes unresponsive and is intubated for airway protection. You contact his family to notify them of the patient's rapidly declining condition.

Question 1

What is this patient's expected mortality at this juncture?

    A. 15%

    B. 25%

    C. 45%

    D. 95%

Question 2

Options for managing this patient at this time include all of the following except:

    A. Intravenous beta-blocking medications to maintain a blood pressure of 120/80 mmHg

    B. Intravenous mannitol to decrease cerebral edema

    C. Intravenous steroids

    D. Right hemicraniectomy and durotomy

Answer 1: C

This patient has suffered a large right middle cerebral artery (MCA) infarction. These types of strokes account for approximately 10–15% of supratentorial infarctions and have a mortality of 50–80%. In one series, 47% of patients died from massive cerebral edema, 6% from non-neurologic causes, and 47% survived at least to day 30 after the stroke. Based upon this study, this patient's expected mortality is around 47% but may be even higher based upon his rapid deterioration.

Answer 2: A

Though this patient's stroke occurred several days ago, hypotension should be avoided. Tight blood pressure control would not be indicated and, if instituted, could lead to hypoperfusion of already compromised areas of brain tissue.

Interestingly, good studies supporting the efficacy of mannitol, steroids, and mechanical hyperventilation are lacking in the medical literature and they have not been shown to improve outcomes. Despite this, there is little evidence that these therapies cause harm, and so they are frequently used for lack of better interventions. This patient received mannitol and mechanical hyperventilation in the ICU. Several days later he had improved and was extubated. Two weeks after admission he was transferred to an acute rehabilitation unit, in stable condition but with persistent left hemiplegia.

Use and timing of hemicraniectomy and durotomy for malignant middle cerebral artery infarction remains controversial in the medical and neurosurgical literature. There is evidence that, in selected populations of patients, hemicraniectomy and durotomy can markedly decrease intracranial pressure and improve short- and intermediate-term outcomes. These procedures involve removing part of the skull and dura. After a minimum of 3 months the stored cranium is then replaced. The best timing of this procedure is unclear, but monitoring for anisocoria as a manifestation of brain-stem herniation, altered level of consciousness, or visualization of right-to-left shift of greater than 1 cm on a CT scan of the brain are sometimes used to determine when to intervene. Studies of this procedure in malignant MCA infarction have been limited by small numbers and heterogeneity of patients being evaluated. Although exact criteria remain to be determined, it does appear that older age and increased number of medical conditions may define a group of patients who do not derive long-term benefit from hemicraniectomy and durotomy.

KASNER S, et al. Predictors of fatal brain edema in massive hemispheric ischemic stroke. *Stroke* 2001;322:117–123.

SCHNECK MJ, ORIGITANO TC. Hemicraniectomy and durotomy for malignant middle cerebral artery infarction. *Neurosurg Clin North Am* 2008;19:459–468.

Case 14

Image contributed by Lailey Oliva

A 45-year-old Vietnamese immigrant is admitted from the Emergency Department (ED) to your service after presenting with 2 days of nausea, vomiting, diarrhea, fever, and mild diffuse abdominal pain. Upon admission her abdomen is soft and nontender, without masses or hepatosplenomegaly. She declines to stand and ambulate due to mild orthostatic dizziness. Musculoskeletal examination reveals obvious atrophy of the left buttock and anterior and lateral thigh musculature. Laboratory testing done in the ED reveals a serum blood urea nitrogen of 4 mg/dL and creatinine of 0.2 mg/dL. A computed tomographic (CT) scan of the abdomen and pelvis does not reveal any abdominal pathology but is remarkable for nearly complete atrophy of the left pelvic girdle (Fig. 14.1) and proximal femur (Fig. 14.2). The patient receives intravenous hydration as well as reassurance. She has no further diarrhea after her arrival at the ED.

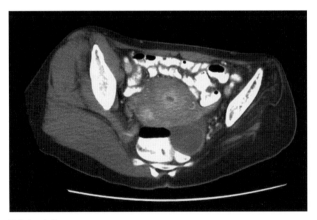

Figure 14.1 Pelvic girdle.

Hospital Images: A Clinical Atlas, First Edition. Edited by Paul B. Aronowitz.
© 2012 Wiley-Blackwell. Published 2012 by John Wiley & Sons, Inc.

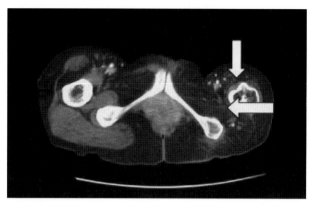

Figure 14.2   Proximal femur.

Question 1

After reviewing the CT scan you return to the patient's bedside to obtain further medical history. This patient is most likely to have had which of the following diseases in the past?

A. *Bordatella pertussis* infection

B. Diphtheria

C. Poliomyelitis

D. Hepatitis B

Question 2

When you arrive at the bedside, the patient's husband expresses concern about whether there will ever be any future complications from this patient's prior disease. Which of the following would you tell him?

A. She will lead a normal, healthy life.

B. She is likely to develop a progressive motor weakness of her lower extremities after the age of 60 that may necessitate use of a wheelchair.

C. She is at significant risk of developing postpolio syndrome, which occurs in more than 80% of polio survivors with significant muscle atrophy.

D. She is at significant risk of developing orthopedic complications from her muscle atrophy, but it is unclear what her risk is of developing further muscle atrophy and weakness.

Answer 1: C

Although this patient could have had any of the listed diseases as a child in Southeast Asia, the one that most likely explains her physical, laboratory, and CT findings is poliomyelitis. Polio is now rare in the United States, and considerable progress has been made in reducing disease burden throughout the world due to increased rates of vaccination. Polio is caused by a small RNA virus classified in the genus *Enterovirus* within the family *Picornaviridae*. It is spread by the fecal–oral route.

While it is believed that 95% of all infections are either asymptomatic or only cause a flulike illness, a small percentage of victims may develop meningitis and a nonparalytic illness. An even smaller percentage develop meningitis and paralytic poliomyelitis. Bulbar paralysis and respiratory failure may also occur. The degree of spinal paralysis and subsequent recovery over months to years can vary tremendously.

This patient's presentation with a presumed gastroenteritis had nothing to do with her remarkable CT findings. She reported a distant history of poliomyelitis while a child in Vietnam and was noted to walk with a slight gait impairment at baseline.

Answer 2: D

This patient is at risk of postpolio syndrome but it is unclear how great that risk is. Postpolio deterioration, years after a patient has been infected with the polio virus, is a somewhat confusing entity. The definition of this disorder varies, with some definitions including complaints of fatigue, pain in muscles and joints, reduced exercise tolerance, and impaired activities of daily living. Others have tried to limit this definition to actual symptomatic postpolio muscular atrophy. It is quite clear that patients with asymmetric muscle atrophy and chronic physical impairment are at increased risk of orthopedic complications due to unusual wear and tear on favored muscles and resultant joint stressors. While the medical literature does not clearly delineate this patient's risk of postpolio syndrome, she is at risk of developing orthopedic complications of her prior disease.

HOWARD RS. Poliomyelitis and the postpolio syndrome. *Brit Med J* 2005;330:1314–1319.
KIDD D, WILLIAMS AJ, HOWARD RS. Poliomyelitis. *Postgrad Med J* 1996;72:641–647.
SOORIASH L. Asymmetric muscle atrophy from childhood polio. *J Hosp Med* 2007;2(6):441.

Case 15

A 42-year-old man with a history of a cadaveric renal transplant for renal failure from polycystic kidney disease is admitted directly to the hospital from his nephrologist's office for complaints of 1 week of profuse, nonbloody diarrhea up to 20 times each day and volume depletion with marked orthostatic pulse and blood pressure changes. He takes immunosuppressive agents due to his renal transplant and reports receiving 10 days of a fluroquinolone antibiotic for a "mild case" of pneumonia 4 months ago. He is ill appearing, with a white blood cell count on admission of 36,000 cells per microliter with 88% neutrophils and 6% bands. Stool cultures for salmonella, shigella, campylobacter, and yersinia are negative. His first *Clostridium difficile* toxin immuonoassay is negative. A colonoscopy is performed (Fig. 15.1).

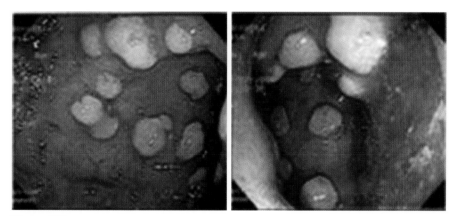

Figure 15.1

Hospital Images: A Clinical Atlas, First Edition. Edited by Paul B. Aronowitz.
© 2012 Wiley-Blackwell. Published 2012 by John Wiley & Sons, Inc.

Question 1

Which of the following would be the best initial therapy in this patient?

    A. Vancomycin 125 mg orally four times a day (QID) for 10–14 days

    B. Metronidazole 500 mg orally three times a day (TID) for 10–14 days

    C. Ciprofloxacin 500 mg orally two times a day (BID) for 10–14 days

    D. Fluconazole 500 mg orally every day (QD) for 4 weeks

Question 2

Regarding this disorder, which of the following is a true statement?

    A. Hand washing with soap and water is not sporicidal but helps reduce its spread.

    B. The Centers for Disease Control and Prevention (CDC) does not recommend the use of barrier precautions.

    C. Alcohol hand sanitizer is sporicidal.

    D. Droplet precautions should be instituted.

Question 3

This patient's chance of recurrence of this disease after initial therapy is approximately:

    A. 2%

    B. 5%

    C. 20%

    D. 50%

Answer 1: A

This image reveals pseudomembrananous colitis, which was confirmed by biopsy. Current expert consensus is that metronidazole can be initiated for mild cases of *Clostridium difficile* infection but that vancomycin should be started for more severe cases. Since this patient is immunocompromised, is volume depleted, appears ill, and has a leukemoid reaction characteristic of more severe cases of *C. difficile* infection, vancomycin should be initiated. If he had been on an antibiotic at the time of admission, it would have been important to stop that agent. It would also have been reasonable to have started empiric treatment based upon his history of antibiotic use. Despite the fact that enzyme immunoassays are good tests, sensitivity can be as low as 75% and sometimes up to three samples must be sent to the laboratory to confirm the diagnosis if the clinician's index of suspicion is high enough.

Broad-spectrum cephalosporins and fluoroquinolones are now the antibiotics most commonly associated with *C. difficile* infection, although any antibiotic exposure can put a patient at risk. Other risk factors include age greater than 65 years, immunocompromised status, hospitalization, residence in a chronic-care facility, gastrointestinal surgery and gastrointestinal procedures, prolonged nasogastric suction, and use of proton pump inhibitors or H_2-blocking agents. Some medical literature indicates that 20–40% of hospitalized patients are colonized with *C. difficile* compared with 2–3% of healthy adults. Complications of *C. difficile* infection can be severe and include toxic megacolon, need for colectomy, hypoalbuminemia, hypovolemic shock, sepsis, acute kidney injury due to volume depletion, and death.

Answer 2: A

Soap and water **do not** kill *C. difficile* spores but the mechanics of hand washing help remove the spores from skin. Alcohol-based hand sanitizers do not kill *C. difficile* spores or remove them. The CDC recommends contact precautions for patients infected with *C. difficile*. *Clostridium difficile* spores are transferred by direct contact and are not aerosolized, and therefore droplet or respiratory precautions should not be instituted.

Answer 3: C

Current rates of recurrence of *C. difficile* infection are approximately 20%. Of this initial relapse group, 55% will have one or more additional relapses. Prior to the year 2000, failure rates with initial treatment were as low as 2–3% but have risen dramatically due the rise of mutated forms of *C. difficile*.

BARTLETT JG. Narrative review: the new epidemic of *Clostridium difficile*–associated enteric disease. *Ann Intern Med* 2006;145:758–764.

CIARÁN KP, LAMONT TJ. *Clostridium difficile*—more difficult than ever. *N Engl J Med* 2008;359(18):1932–1940.

Case 16

You are called to consult on a 76-year-old woman who fell and broke her hip while stepping onto a bus. The orthopedic surgeon is concerned about an abnormal blood count. Other than hip pain she is asymptomatic and was independent in all of her activities at home. She does not have any lymphadenopathy or hepatic or splenic enlargement. Her white blood cell count (WBC) is 24,000 cells per microliter. Differential blood count reveals 88% lymphocytes. Her blood smear is shown in Figure 16.1.

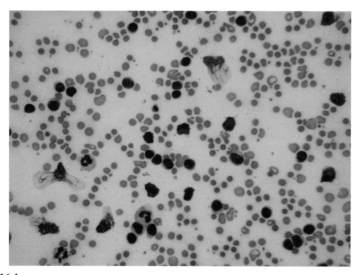

Figure 16.1

Hospital Images: A Clinical Atlas, First Edition. Edited by Paul B. Aronowitz.
© 2012 Wiley-Blackwell. Published 2012 by John Wiley & Sons, Inc.

Question 1

Which of the following statements is correct?

    A. Surgery should be postponed and the patient should be seen by a hematologist for evaluation and initiation of chemotherapy.

    B. The most common infectious complications of this disease are meningitis and septic arthritis.

    C. This disease is usually discovered incidentally in elderly patients.

    D. This is a disease characterized by abnormal T-cell proliferation.

    E. This is an uncommon disease.

Later in the evening the patient's husband asks to speak with you. He asks you what his wife's prognosis is, based on her hematologic abnormality.

Question 2

You would tell the patient's husband that her approximate chance of survival is:

    A. 10% at 5 years

    B. 25% at 5 years

    C. 75% at 5 years

    D. Unlikely beyond 6 months

Question 3

Future complications of this disease might include which of the following:

    A. Conversion to acute myelogenous leukemia (AML)

    B. Conversion to acute lymphoblastic leukemia (ALL)

    C. Conversion to acute lymphoblastic lymphoma

    D. Hemolytic anemia

    E. Both C and D

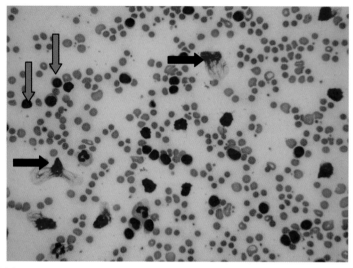

Figure 16.2

Answer 1: C

This case illustrates a classic presentation of chronic lymphocytic leukemia (CLL)—the most common leukemia in the Western world. The majority of patients presenting with this disease are older than 60 years, and more than 50% of diagnoses are made incidentally. CLL is a B-cell leukemia manifested by relatively large numbers of mature B lymphocytes. This patient's blood smear (Fig. 16.2) shows small mature lymphocytes (light arrows) and "smudge cells" (black arrows). Mature lymphocytes are normally small and have nucleoli that occupy most of the cell's cytoplasm as in this case. Smudge cells appear during the preparation of the smear, as the leukemic B cells have relatively fragile cell membranes and are easily damaged (smudged) during processing.

The most common infectious complications of CLL are increased rates of community-acquired pneumonia and sinusitis; this is thought to be secondary to a dysfunctional immune system.

Answer 2: C

In the absence of lymphadenopathy, fevers, weight loss, hepatomegaly, or splenomegaly this patient has a good prognosis, which is approximately 75% at 5 years.

Answer 3: E

Although relatively uncommon, there are a few important complications that may occur in patients with CLL. Conversion to acute lymphoblastic lymphoma, also known as Richter syndrome, occurs in less than 10% of patients with CLL. Patients with CLL may also develop a warm antibody (immunoglobulin G [IgG]) hemolytic anemia that is usually responsive to corticosteroid therapy. The main clue seen on the blood smear for hemolytic anemia would be spherocytes. Spherocytes are formed as the red blood cell membrane is stripped passing through the spleen due to immunoglobulin bound to the membrane.

Case 17

A 56-year-old man is admitted to your service for fevers of 2 weeks' duration. The nurse practitioner you are supervising calls you to examine the patient's fingers (Fig. 17.1).

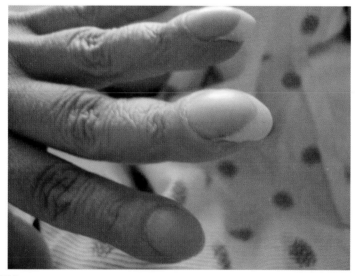

Figure 17.1

Hospital Images: A Clinical Atlas, First Edition. Edited by Paul B. Aronowitz.
© 2012 Wiley-Blackwell. Published 2012 by John Wiley & Sons, Inc.

Question 1

Which of the following is the only disease that you would *not* consider as a possible cause of this finding?

A. Endocarditis

B. Cirrhosis

C. Chronic obstructive pulmonary disease

D. Cyanotic congenital heart disease

E. Interstitial pulmonary fibrosis

Question 2

While examining the patient with the nurse practitioner, she asks you whether you think his toes are "abnormal" (Fig. 17.2). Which of the following would you tell her?

A. The patient's toes are normal.

B. The patient has koilonychia.

C. The patient's toes are also clubbed.

D. The patient has splinter hemorrhages of his toenails.

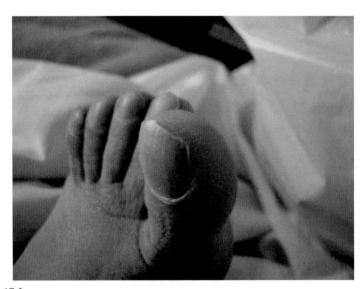

Figure 17.2

Answer 1: C

Chronic obstructive pulmonary disease does not cause clubbing. However, there are many diseases that are associated with clubbing. This patient has had clubbing since childhood, when he was diagnosed with cyanotic congenital heart disease from tetralogy of Fallot. There are various methods of examining the fingers for the presence of clubbing. Physical examination will reveal the presence of sponginess of the finger just proximal to the cuticle, an increase in the nail fold convexity, and thickening of the distal phalange causing greater distal phalangeal depth compared with the distal interphalangeal joint—normally the opposite.

   The mechanism of clubbing is not clear but recent medical literature has indicated that vascular endothelial growth factor (VEGF), a platelet-derived factor induced by hypoxia or inflammation, may play a role in digital clubbing. Processes that alter normal pulmonary circulation disrupt fragmentation of megakaryocytes in the lung into platelets. Whole megakaryocytes enter the systemic circulation and become impacted in the peripheral capillaries, where they cause local tissue hypoxia and the release of platelet-derived growth factor and VEGF, leading to the vascular hyperplasia that underlies clubbing.

Answer 2: C

This patient's toes are also clubbed. Koilonychia is spooning of the nails that results from chronic iron-deficiency anemia. Splinter hemorrhages may occur with subacute bacterial endocarditis but are not seen in this patient's toenails.

MARTINEZ-LAVIN M. Exploring the cause of the most ancient clinical sign of medicine: finger clubbing. *Semin Arth Rheum* 2007;36:380–385.

NGUYEN K, ARONOWITZ P. Drumstick digits: a case of clubbing of the fingers and toes. *J Hosp Med* 2010;5(3):196.

SPICKNALL KE, ZIRWAS MJ, ENGLISH JC. Clubbing: an update on diagnosis, differential diagnosis, pathophysiology, and clinical relevance. *J Am Acad Dermatol* 2005;52:1020–1028.

Case 18

Image contributed by David Jacobson

An 83-year-old Asian man with a history of dementia is being admitted to your service for community-acquired pneumonia. Due to the patient's dementia, he is unable to provide meaningful medical history. The third-year medical student contacts you while seeing the patient in the Emergency Department. The student is concerned that the patient's family may be abusing him and asks whether he should call Adult Protective Services to initiate an investigation. On physical examination the patient has a fever of 38.6°C, rales present at the right, posterior, lower chest on auscultation, and rounded skin lesions (Fig. 18.1).

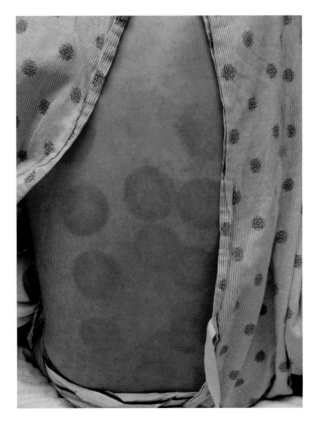

Figure 18.1

Hospital Images: A Clinical Atlas, First Edition. Edited by Paul B. Aronowitz.
© 2012 Wiley-Blackwell. Published 2012 by John Wiley & Sons, Inc.

Question

Which of the following would you tell the student to do?

- **A.** Contact Social Work and Adult Protective Services.
- **B.** Check stat fibrinogen, prothrombin time (PT), partial thromboplastin time (PTT), and fibrin split products to evaluate for disseminated intravascular coagulation (DIC).
- **C.** Reassure the student and advise him not to contact Adult Protective Services.
- **D.** Advise him not to contact Adult Protective Services and to educate the patient's family about proper use of heating pads.

Answer: C

This patient has been treated with cupping. The mechanism of cupping involves application of a vacuum to a closed, inverted cup system applied to an area of the skin. The vacuum causes disruption of superficial capillaries, which results in redness, petechiae, and ecchymosis. Cupping therapy is a popular technique in traditional Chinese medicine and so it is important to be aware of its use among immigrants from Asian countries, particularly China and Vietnam. Cupping and coining (the use of coins to agitate the skin) may be confused with child or elder abuse so obtaining a detailed medical history, in the presence of an experienced translator, is important in order to avoid confusion. While cupping is frequently associated with traditional Chinese medicine, it was also used in ancient Egypt, by Hippocrates in ancient Greece, and by Zulu physicians in Africa. Instruments used to perform cupping have evolved from bull and other animal horns in ancient times to plastic or glass cups today. Western physicians utilized cupping, leeches, and scarification until modern times. George Orwell, the well-known English writer, described his treatment for pneumonia in a Paris hospital in 1929 as involving cupping glasses, scarification, and mustard poultice.

LIN CW, et al. Iatrogenic bullae following cupping therapy. *J Altern Complement Med* 2009;15(11): 1243–1245.

UNDERWOOD EA. Bleeding, cupping and purging. *Brit Med J* 1955:42–43.

WONG GHC, WONG JKT, WONG NYY. Signs of physical abuse or evidence of moxibustion, cupping or coining? *Can Med Assoc J* 1999;160(6):785–786.

Case 19

Written by Nicole Gonzales

An 81-year-old man presents to the Emergency Department with a 3-month history of progressively worsening nonproductive cough, fatigue, night sweats, and 10-lb weight loss. He does not smoke and has a ranch in Arizona that he visits several times per year. He recently completed a 10-day course of an advanced fluoroquinolone antibiotic prescribed by his primary care physician, but his symptoms continued to worsen despite this therapy. Chest radiograph shows a left lung infiltrate (arrow, Fig. 19.1).

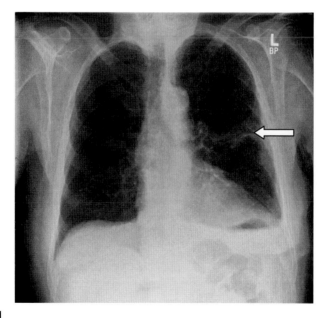

Figure 19.1

Hospital Images: A Clinical Atlas, First Edition. Edited by Paul B. Aronowitz.
© 2012 Wiley-Blackwell. Published 2012 by John Wiley & Sons, Inc.

Question 1

Which of the following is the most appropriate treatment for this patient?

    A. Regular monitoring as an outpatient; no other treatment for now

    B. Fluconazole 200 mg daily for 1 month

    C. Fluconazole 400 mg daily for 3–6 months

    D. Fluconazole 400 mg daily for 1 year

    E. Fluconazole 200 mg daily, lifelong treatment

Question 2

Which of the following would provide the most helpful information about this patient's prognosis?

    A. Culture positivity

    B. Serologic testing with enzyme immunoassay (EIA)

    C. Complement fixation titers

    D. Biopsy with special stains and culture

Answer 1: D

This patient has coccidioidomycosis, causing chronic progressive fibrocavitary pneumonia. It is caused by *Coccidioides immitis*, which has a two-phase life cycle. The organism initially exists in soil in the mycelial phase as a mold, growing in branching, septate hyphae. After rain, it multiplies and forms arthrocondia. After dispersion by wind and inhalation by the host, it progresses into the spherule phase in the lung. Spherules are multinucleated spherical structures containing endospores (Fig. 19.2). Eventually the spherules break open and release endospores. Each endospore goes on to form a new spherule.

Coccidioidomycosis is common in the Southwestern United States, California's Central Valley, and some areas in northern Mexico, where the climate includes hot summers, mild winters, and less than 20 inches of rainfall per year. This incidence increases further when rainy summers are followed by dry winters and windstorms.

Clinically, coccidioidomycosis can present in several forms, including acute pneumonia, chronic progressive pneumonia, pulmonary nodules and cavities, extrapulmonary nonmeningeal disease, and meningitis. Acute pneumonia usually occurs 1–3 weeks following inhalation of the organism, and presenting symptoms are similar to community-acquired pneumonia, including cough and fatigue. Symptoms of headache and pleuritic pain can suggest coccidioidomycosis. Hilar and paratracheal adenopathy is also present on chest X-rays in 25% of coccidioidal infections. Many cases resolve without treatment. Diffuse pneumonia, showing up as small, diffuse nodules throughout both lungs, is more common in immunocompromised hosts or those who have inhaled a large number of spores.

Chronic progressive pneumonia (as in this patient) occurs in a small percentage of patients and is characterized by persistent illness lasting more than 3 months. These patients can suffer from persistent, productive cough, hemoptysis, and weight loss. Dense unifocal or multifocal consolidations form and can include areas of consolidation.

Extrapulmonary disease usually occurs in the immunocompromised, but it occurs in less than 5% of immunocompetent hosts. This form of the disease may occur in the skin, lymph

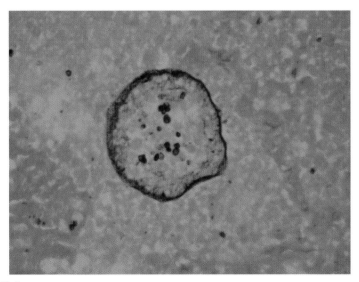

Figure 19.2

nodes, bones, and joints. Meningitis can be catastrophic with severe long-term morbidity, even when identified and treated appropriately. Patients with cerebral infarction or hydrocephalus have the highest mortality rate.

Treatment depends on the severity of disease. Acute pneumonia usually resolves without treatment in immunocompetent hosts. Treatment is recommended for those in their third trimester of pregnancy and should be considered in people of African or Filipino descent (who have higher risk of severe infection) or in people who are more severely ill. Treatment consists of oral azole antifungal agents at 200–400 mg/day for 3–6 months. In cases of chronic progressive fibrocavitary pneumonia, treatment is recommended with oral azole antifungal agents for 1 year. If the patient does not respond to therapy, an alternative azole or amphotericin B should be used. Disseminated pneumonia should be treated with amphotericin B or high-dose fluconazole, for a total duration of 1 year. Immunocompromised patients should remain on azole antifungal therapy indefinitely.

Answer 2: C

Diagnosis of coccidioidomycosis requires one of the following:

1. Identification of coccidioides spherules in cytology or biopsy
2. A positive culture from any body fluid
3. Positive serologic testing

Positive cultures always indicate infection, as *Coccidioides* is not a colonizing species. Cultures are rarely positive, so serologic studies should always be ordered. Serologic testing seeks immunoglobulin IgM and IgG antibodies to *Coccidioides* antigen. This can be done by immunodiffusion, EIA, or counterimmunoelectrophoresis, which are qualitative methods. Complement fixation is a quantitative measurement of IgG and can provide prognostic information, a lower titer indicating a more favorable prognosis. A complement fixation titer of 1:16 or greater indicates more severe illness. Serial testing can also provide information about response to treatment.

GALGIANI JN, et al. IDSA Guidelines: coccidioidomycosis. *Clin Infect Dis* 2005;41:1217–1223.
PARISH B. Coccidioidomycosis. *Mayo Clin Proc* 2008;83(3):343–349.

Case 20

Image contributed by Niraj Seghal and Bob Wachter

A 62-year-old man is transferred to your medical center for neurosurgical evaluation for a complicated epidural abscess. As you enter the patient's room, the third-year resident, an intern, and a medical student are discussing the patient's color-coded wristbands (Fig. 20.1). They ask you if you know what all of his color-coded wristbands signify since the patient is unsure what they mean.

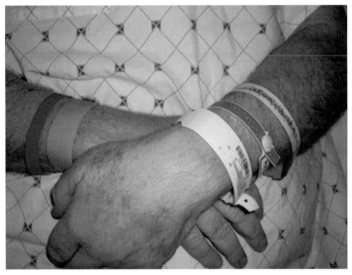

Figure 20.1   Color-coded wristbands (left-to-right: purple, green, white, red, and yellow).

Hospital Images: A Clinical Atlas, First Edition. Edited by Paul B. Aronowitz.
© 2012 Wiley-Blackwell. Published 2012 by John Wiley & Sons, Inc.

Question

You would tell them that the white band is definitely his patient identifier, and you would also tell them which of the following:

A. Purple means "Do Not Resuscitate"; yellow, he is a fall risk; green, he is allergic to tape; and red, he has at least one medication allergy.

B. Purple means he is a fall risk; yellow, Do Not Resuscitate; red, he has a medication allergy; and green, he is confused.

C. Yellow is a Lance Armstrong "Live Strong" wristband; purple means Do Not Resuscitate; green, he has a tape allergy; and red, he has a medication allergy.

D. You aren't sure what all the colors mean since attempts to standardize color-coded wristbands have been inconsistent across the American health-care system.

Answer: D

Although the primary team accepting this patient was able to clarify that the green band represented fall risk, purple meant a tape allergy, and red indicated a medication allergy, they were unable to clarify what the yellow wristband signified. While the use of color-coded wristbands has risen in an attempt to improve patient safety, the lack of standardization throughout the United States and Great Britain has contributed to confusion in patient care. One study in Great Britain found that 4 different colors were being used by different hospitals to signify risk of fall and the color red was being used for 10 different statuses or risks. Participants surveyed at individual hospitals were not always sure whether color-coded wristbands were being used in their hospitals and when they knew they were not always sure what the colors represented.

A 2006 survey of nurse executives done in California found that 7 solid colors and various multicolored bands were being used to represent 29 different conditions in California hospitals. Results of a nursing survey carried out in Missouri hospitals and long-term care facilities and published in 2007 found that 29 different colors were being used to communicate 21 different clinical conditions. The American Hospital Association has endorsed the use of purple wristbands to represent "Do Not Resuscitate," yellow for fall risk, and red for allergies. As of 2008, the Joint Commission, the leading accreditation agency in the United States, expressed caution about this system. Numerous hospitals have been reluctant to openly tag patient "code status" due to privacy concerns as well as concern surrounding the subtleties of interpretation surrounding the term "Do Not Resuscitate." Other hospitals have added "DNR" labeling to the purple wristbands to more clearly delineate the meaning of purple.

Some authors in Great Britain have advised that, other than the standard white wristband containing patient identification information, a red band be used to alert health-care providers that there is at least one significant patient issue and that these issues should be sought out in the patient's medical record. Remarkably, despite their frequent use, it remains unclear whether color-coded wristbands actually improve patient safety.

The best approach in this patient's care would have been to re-evaluate each of his risks or statuses and to remove wristbands that were confusing or contradictory to the color coding in use at the receiving hospital.

ANANNY L. Colour-coded wristbands confusing. *Can Med Assoc J* 2009;180(2);161.

CIZEK KE, et al. A crystal-clear call to standardize color-coded wristbands. *Nursing* 2010;40(5):57–59.

SEGHAL N, WACHTER RM. Color coded wrist bands: promoting safety or confusion? *J Hosp Med* 2007;2(6):445.

SEGHAL N, WACHTER RM. Identification of inpatient DNR status: a safety hazard begging for standardization. *J Hosp Med* 2007;2(6):366–371.

SEVDALIS N, et al. Designing evidence-based patient safety interventions: the case of the UK's National Health Service hospital wristbands. *J Eval Clin Pract* 2009;15:316–322.

Case 21

Images contributed by Julie Gillespie Payne

A 62-year-old man with a history of coronary artery disease and placement of two drug-eluting coronary stents 5 months ago and prostate cancer previously treated with total prostatectomy presents with 6 weeks of progressively worsening dyspnea when climbing stairs and lower extremity edema. He denies fever, chills, sweats, weight loss, or recent upper respiratory tract infections. No one is ill in his home. The patient is seen by his cardiologist and an electrocardiogram done in his office reveals new nonspecific ST-segment changes in the precordial leads. Because of concern that the patient may have unstable angina due to stent occlusion, the patient is admitted directly to the cardiac cathetherization laboratory. Catheterization reveals that coronary stents have good flow and that cardiac function is normal. A right heart catheterization reveals equalization of diastolic pressures in the right atrium, right ventricle, left ventricle, left atrium, and pulmonary capillary bed. The patient is admitted to the cardiology service and you are consulted for input on medical therapy.

Your physical examination reveals a pleasant patient in no distress. His lungs are clear to auscultation, but there are slightly decreased breath sounds at the bases with dullness to percussion. His jugular venous pulse is elevated to the angle of the jaw but he does not have any extra heart sounds or murmurs. He has pitting edema up to his knees. A chest radiograph and computed tomographic (CT) scan of the chest are obtained (Figs. 21.1 and 21.2).

Hospital Images: A Clinical Atlas, First Edition. Edited by Paul B. Aronowitz.
© 2012 Wiley-Blackwell. Published 2012 by John Wiley & Sons, Inc.

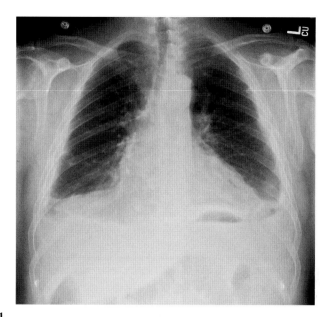

Figure 21.1

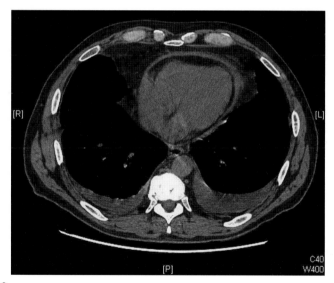

Figure 21.2

Question 1

What is the best subsequent step in this patient's management?

    A. Administer furosemide 80 mg intravenously twice per day and monitor for improvement.

    B. Begin nonsteroidal anti-inflammatory drug (NSAID) therapy with close follow-up.

C. Initiate angiotensin converting enzyme (ACE) inhibitor therapy.

D. Urgent cardiothoracic surgery consultation for pericardiectomy.

E. Tuberculosis skin testing (PPD) and empiric initiation of four-drug antituberculous medications.

On hospital day number 2 the patient is quite anxious. With his wife and daughter at the bedside he tells you he is worried that he has cancer and wants to know what you think.

Question 2

You would tell him that he probably does not have cancer and that the most likely cause of his disorder is:

A. Tuberculosis

B. Autoimmune disease

C. His previous cardiac stenting procedure

D. Viral pericarditis

Answer 1: B

The findings on this patient's chest X-ray (bilateral pleural effusions; Fig. 21.3, arrows) and CT scan (thickened pericardium; Fig. 21.4, arrow) are classic for constrictive pericarditis. Assuming the cause to be a recent viral pericaditis, initial treatment in this setting could include NSAID or colchicine therapy with very close follow-up after discharge. If there is no improvement on anti-inflammatory medications or worsening over the next 3 months, peri-cardiectomy should be considered. Consultation should be obtained from cardiothoracic surgery while the patient is still in the hospital. Since the mortality from pericardiectomy is as high as 6% in medical centers experienced in this procedure, conservative therapy is ini-tially recommended.

Although diuretics might help diminish this patient's dyspnea on exertion and edema, administration should be done cautiously. An intravenous dose of 80 mg (equivalent to 160 mg orally) given twice each day to a patient who is "naïve" to diuretics could precipitously drop filling pressures. These patients tend to be very pre-load dependent and overly aggressive diuresis could reduce cardiac output, causing orthostatic hypotension, dizziness, or even syncope. This patient has normal cardiac function so an ACE inhibitor would not be indicated. A PPD should be placed since tuberculosis is a common cause of constrictive pericarditis throughout the world. Since tuberculosis is a less common cause of constrictive pericarditis in the United States and there are no other signs of active tuberculosis, antituberculous medi-cations would not be indicated at this time.

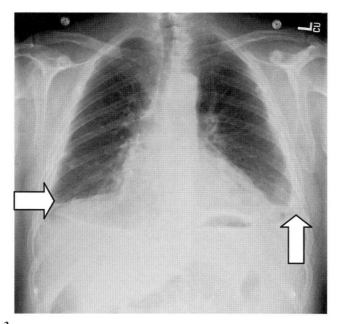

Figure 21.3

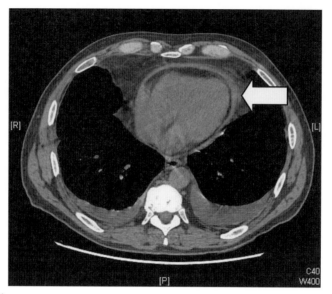

Figure 21.4

Answer 2: D

Prior mantle radiation, previous cardiothoracic surgery, and viral pericarditis are leading causes of constrictive pericarditis in the United States. Tuberculosis and connective tissue diseases should also be considered. Since this patient did not have a history of prior cardiothoracic surgery or radiation therapy, the most likely etiology of his disorder would be viral pericarditis. A PPD should be placed and the patient's blood tested for the presence of antinuclear antibodies and rheumatoid factor. An uncomplicated cardiac catheterization with or without coronary stenting does not cause constrictive pericarditis.

CRANDALL MA, MULVAGH SL. 68-year-old woman with chronic cough and recurrent pleural effusions. *Mayo Clin Proc* 2010;85(5):479–482.

KHANDAKER MH, et al. Pericardial disease: diagnosis and management. *Mayo Clin Proc* 2010; 85(6):572–593.

NISHIMURA RA. Constrictive pericarditis in the modern era: a diagnostic dilemma. *Heart* 2001; 86:619–623.

Case **22**

Image contributed by Cleon Yee

A 58-year-old man presents to the Emergency Department for diffuse abdominal pain, nausea, and two episodes of emesis. His vital signs are stable and his abdominal examination reveals high-pitched bowel sounds and abdominal distension with mild, diffuse tenderness. An upright abdominal X-ray (Fig. 22.1) reveals multiple foreign bodies and air fluid levels.

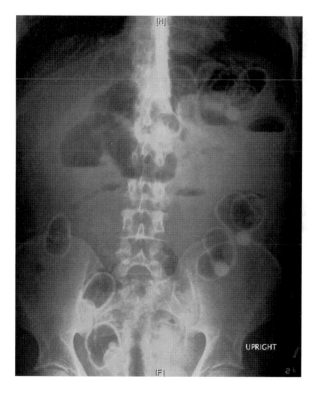

Figure 22.1

Hospital Images: A Clinical Atlas, First Edition. Edited by Paul B. Aronowitz.
© 2012 Wiley-Blackwell. Published 2012 by John Wiley & Sons, Inc.

Question

The most likely etiology of these foreign bodies is ingestion of which of the following:

   A. Cocaine packets
   B. Lithium batteries
   C. Dolls' heads
   D. Paper clips

Answer: C

Although accidental ingestion of foreign bodies is a relatively common problem in the pediatric population, ingestion of foreign bodies is almost always voluntary in adults. While accidental ingestion of foreign bodies in adults tends to occur in elderly patients or patients under the influence of alcohol, voluntary ingestion occurs due to psychiatric illness or attempts to smuggle or hide illicit objects or drugs. Deliberate ingestion of foreign bodies is common among prison inmates.

Although the physician seeing this patient would consider "body packing," the carrying of illicit drugs wrapped in condoms, the X-ray appearance is not typical. There is usually a "double condom" sign, where air is present between two condoms and the center of the foreign body would be more radio dense than in this image. As seen in a different patient (Fig. 22.2), paperclips (thin arrow) and batteries (thick arrow) have a different appearance than dolls' heads. Additional medical history would also be helpful to clarify the type of ingestion.

In this patient further history revealed that this patient had an oral and anal fetish revolving around the ingestion of dolls' heads. After experiencing a similar dolls'-head-related bowel obstruction 20 years previously, he had learned to manufacture his own dolls' heads so that they passed through the ileocecal valve without difficulty. On this occasion, he required a laparotomy to remove the dolls' heads and had an unremarkable recovery.

Plain radiographs are usually the first step in the initial evaluation of a patient suspected of ingesting a foreign body. Fifty percent of children with confirmed foreign body ingestions are asymptomatic. The size, shape, and number of foreign bodies is not predictive of the ability to transit the gastrointestinal tract. While some literature suggests that most ingested

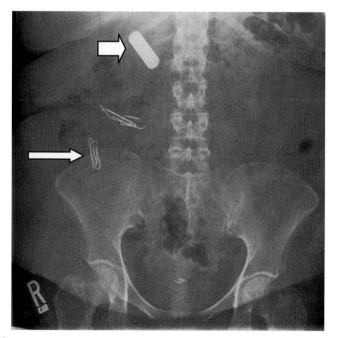

Figure 22.2

foreign bodies will pass spontaneously, some retrospective studies have shown an intervention rate of as high as 36% in a Northern Ireland prison population.

ARANA A, et al. Management of ingested foreign bodies in childhood and review of the literature. *Eur J Pediatr* 2001;160:468–472.

BISHARAT M, et al. Foreign body ingestion in prisoners—the Belfast experience. *Ulster Med J* 2008;77(2);110–114.

TRAUB SJ, HOFFMAN RS, NELSON LS. Body packing—the internal concealment of illicit drugs. *N Engl J Med* 2003;349(26):2519–2526.

WEILAND ST, SCHURR MJ. Conservative management of ingested foreign bodies. *J Gastrointest Surg* 2002;6(3):496–500.

Case 23

Written by Vanessa London

Images contributed by Vanessa London and David Peng

A 35-year-old man presents to the Emergency Department (ED) with a 3-day history of a diffuse, morbilliform rash. Due to a history of a childhood seizure, he was recently begun on phenytoin by his primary care physician. Three weeks later, he noted fever, abdominal pain, and nausea, followed by the development of a rash. His physical examination reveals an oral temperature of 38.2°C, cervical lymphadenopathy, and a diffuse, morbilliform rash (Fig. 23.1 and Fig. 23.2). Laboratory testing shows a white blood cell count of 16,000 cells per microliter, with 66%

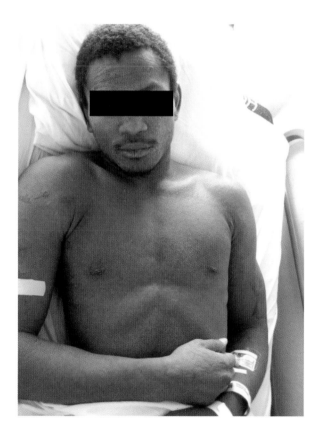

Figure 23.1

Hospital Images: A Clinical Atlas, First Edition. Edited by Paul B. Aronowitz.
© 2012 Wiley-Blackwell. Published 2012 by John Wiley & Sons, Inc.

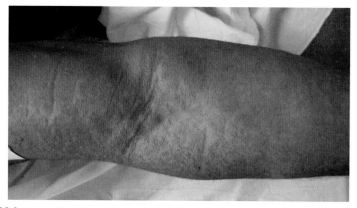

Figure 23.2 Right forearm.

lymphocytes, 25% eosinophils, and 9% neutrophils, and aspartate aminotransferase (AST) 1135 IU/L and alanine aminotransferase (ALT) 850 IU/L.

Question

The most likely diagnosis is which of the following:

    A. Viral exanthema

    B. Stevens–Johnson syndrome

    C. Lymphoma

    D. Drug reaction with eosinophilia and systemic symptoms (DRESS)

    E. Serum sickness

Answer: D

Drug reaction with eosinophilia and systemic symptoms (DRESS) is a life-threatening reaction characterized by fever, skin rash, lymphocytosis with eosinophilia or atypical lymphocytes, lymphadenopathy, and liver or renal dysfunction. Hepatomegaly and splenomegaly may be present on physical examination. Mortality is about 10% and is usually attributed to liver failure, renal failure, or interstitial pneumonitis. Antiepileptic drugs are the most common etiology of DRESS and this reaction is thought to occur in 1 of 1000–10,000 exposures. There are many different names for similar drug reactions, such as anticonvulsant hypersensitivity syndrome, phenytoin syndrome, dapsone syndrome, and allopurinol hypersensitivity syndrome. It has been proposed that DRESS should be used to encompass any of these drug reactions with the characteristic systemic findings.

KANO Y, SHIOHARA T. The variable clinical picture of drug-induced hypersensitivity syndrome/drug rash with eosinophilia and systemic symptoms in relation to the eliciting drug. *Immunol Allergy Clin North Am* 2009;29(3):481–501.

Case 24

A 23-year-old man with a history of asthma and eczema is admitted to the hospital from his dermatologist's office to your service for fever, malaise, and a diffuse rash (Fig. 24.1) with widespread vesicles (Fig. 24.2) and crusted lesions. The rash began 48 hours prior to admission and is mildly pruritic. A Tzanck smear performed in the dermatologist's office shows multinucleated giant cells, and bacterial and viral cultures of the vesicular lesions have been collected and are pending.

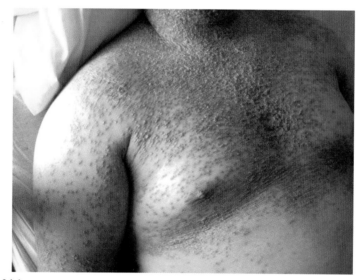

Figure 24.1

Hospital Images: A Clinical Atlas, First Edition. Edited by Paul B. Aronowitz.
© 2012 Wiley-Blackwell. Published 2012 by John Wiley & Sons, Inc.

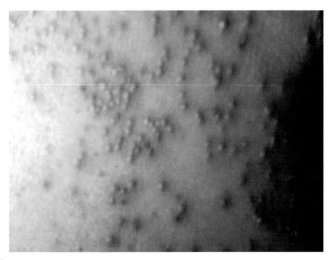

Figure 24.2

Question

This patient has which of the following:

    A. Eczema herpeticum

    B. Staphylococcal scalded skin syndrome

    C. Secondary syphilis

    D. Drug reaction with eosinophilia and systemic symptoms (DRESS)

Answer: A

This patient has eczema herpeticum, also known as herpes simplex virus–associated Kaposi varicelliform eruption. This disorder occurs when eczematous lesions become secondarily infected with herpes simplex virus type 1 or type 2. Viral and bacterial cultures of the vesicles should be sent and the patient started on oral or intravenous acyclovir. This patient responded to oral acyclovir and was discharged home in 72 hours after rapid improvement in his skin lesions. The mortality from eczema herpeticum prior to the development of acyclovir was previously as high as 9%.

These lesions are not characteristic of staphylococcal scalded skin syndrome; however, staphylococcal folliculitis will have pink papules and pustules centered around hair follicles. The diffuse appearance of this patient's rash makes folliculitis an unlikely diagnosis. Secondary syphilis is usually a diffuse macular or maculopapular rash, which is frequently present on the palms of the hands and the soles of the feet. Vesicles would not be consistent with secondary syphilis. DRESS occurs in association with medication ingestion and we are not told whether this patient is taking any medications or whether he has eosinophilia or other systemic symptoms such as fever.

Guss DA. Eczema herpeticum (Images in Emergency Medicine). *Ann Emer Med* 2008;52(1):83.
Treadwell PA. Eczema and infection. *Pediatr Infect Dis J* 2008;27(6):551–552.

Case 25

Images contributed by Ernie Lo, Mike Ren, and Peter Hui

A 65-year-old man with a history of tobacco use, chronic obstructive pulmonary disease, and a recently discovered right lung nodule presents to the Emergency Department (ED) due to shortness of breath and dyspnea on exertion. On physical examination he appears mildly tachypneic but in no distress, with a respiratory rate of 28, blood pressure 100/60 mmHg, and pulse 130 beats per minute. His lungs are clear to auscultation and his cardiac examination shows jugular venous distension 15 cm above the right atrium and distant heart sounds.

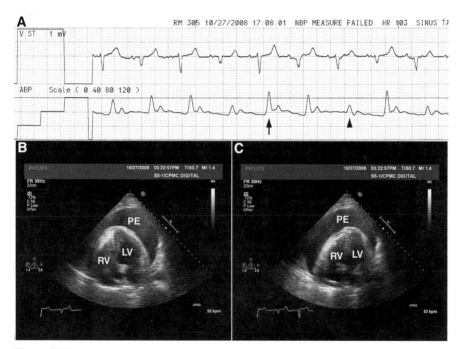

Figure 25.1 (A) Cardiac rhythm (top line) and systolic blood pressure (bottom line); (B,C) echocardiogram (LV, left ventricle; RV, right ventricle; PE, pericardial effusion).

Hospital Images: A Clinical Atlas, First Edition. Edited by Paul B. Aronowitz.
© 2012 Wiley-Blackwell. Published 2012 by John Wiley & Sons, Inc.

Question 1

Which of the following is the variation in electrical activity in the rhythm strip (Fig. 25.1A, top line) called?

A. Pulsus alternans

B. Situs inversus

C. Electrical alternans

D. Alternating ectopy

Due to worsening hypotension shortly after admission to the Cardiac Care Unit, an arterial line is placed (Fig. 25.1A, bottom line). The systolic blood pressure varies from 136 mmHg (arrow) to 96 mmHg (arrowhead). An echocardiogram is shown in the lower images (Fig. 25.1B,C).

Question 2

Which of the following is the explanation for the marked variation in blood pressure in this patient?

A. Increased filling of the right ventricle during inspiration, with resultant decreased left ventricular filling and cardiac output

B. Cardiac ischemia

C. Increased filling of the right ventricle during expiration, with resultant decreased left ventricular filling and cardiac output

D. Massive pulmonary embolus

Question 3

Which of the following is the *least* sensitive finding for this patient's acute medical problem?

A. Tachycardia

B. Diminished heart sounds

C. Elevated jugular venous pulse

D. Pulsus paradoxus

Question 4

What is the best subsequent step in this patient's management?

A. Consult a cardiothoracic surgeon for pericardiectomy.

B. Administer thrombolytic agents.

C. Perform pericardiocentesis.

D. Administer intravenous fluids and nonsteroidal anti-inflammatory drugs, and test for anti-nuclear antibodies and rheumatoid factor.

Answer 1: C

Electrical alternans occurs as the heart swings within a large fluid-filled pericardial sac. Electrical forces change or alternate as the heart moves toward and then away from ("swinging heart"—see Fig. 25.1B,C) electrocardiographic leads.

Answer 2: A

Pulsus paradoxus is believed to occur due to increased filling of the right ventricle during inspiration, with bowing of the ventricular septum and resultant decreased left ventricular filling and cardiac output. Both chambers are limited by the pericardial effusion (PE; Fig. 25.1B,C). Negative intrapleural pressures during inspiration cause increased right ventricular filling and septal bowing into the left ventricle. Septal bowing leads to less filling of the left ventricle, decreasing cardiac output, resulting in a decrease in systolic blood pressure. This finding can also be checked by palpating the pulse and noting a respiratory diminution of the pulse. This dimished pulse is a normal physiologic response but is increased when there is a pericardial effusion of significant size, due to compression of the heart. This finding is best appreciated by inflating a blood pressure cuff and listening to the Korotkoff sounds. Initially these sounds are intermittent, present during expiration but absent during inspiration. As the cuff is deflated the sounds become audible throughout inspiration as well as expiration. The difference in the blood pressure between where they are first audible and where they are audible throughout the respiratory cycle is noted. In normal "physiologic" states, this difference is less than 10 mmHg. If this difference is greater than 10 mmHg, it is considered pulsus paradoxus. An arterial line is a more accurate way to measure this blood pressure difference. In this case the pulsus paradoxus was 40 mmHg (136 minus 96 equals 40).

Answer 3: B

This patient has cardiac tamponade. The pooled sensitivity for the physicial finding of diminished heart sounds is only 24%. More sensitive physical findings include pulsus paradoxus greater than 10 mmHg (82%), tachycardia (77%), and elevated jugular venous pulse 76%.

Answer 4: C

This patient is symptomatic and hypotensive, so a pericardiocentesis should be carried out; 1100 cc of bloody pericardial fluid was removed and the patient was subsequently diagnosed with lung cancer with metastatic disease of the pericardium.

Pericardiectomy would not be a treatment in this condition; however, depending on availability, a cardiothoracic surgeon could be consulted for urgent pericardial drainage and placement of a pericardial window in lieu of a pericardiocentesis. Thrombolytics are a potential treatment for patients with hemodynamically significant pulmonary emboli. NSAIDs are a treatment for viral, autoimmune, or idiopathic pericarditis but not for pericardial tamponade from cancer metastatic to the pericardium.

HOIT BD. Pericardial disease and pericardial tamponade. *Crit Care Med* 2007;35(8):S355-S364.

LO E, REN X, HUI PY. Electrical alternans and pulsus paradoxus. *J Hosp Med* 2010;5(4):253–254.

ROY CL, et al. Does this patient with a pericardial effusion have cardiac tamponade? *JAMA* 2007;297(16):1810–1818.

Case 26

Image contributed by Cam-Tu Tran

A 16-year-old male Cambodian immigrant presents to the Emergency Department with complaints of several weeks of increasing abdominal girth, lower extremity edema, and increasing fatigue (Fig. 26.1). His family says that he was diagnosed with a heart murmur at an early age and that he was told he would eventually need heart surgery or his heart would "fail."

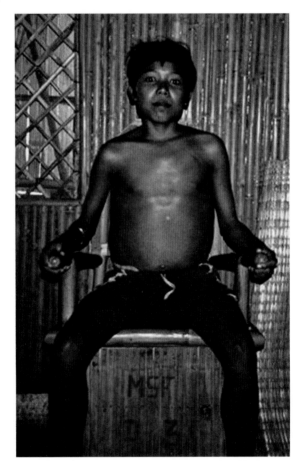

Figure 26.1

Hospital Images: A Clinical Atlas, First Edition. Edited by Paul B. Aronowitz.
© 2012 Wiley-Blackwell. Published 2012 by John Wiley & Sons, Inc.

Question

Which of the following statements is most accurate regarding this boy's most prominent physical findings?

A. His stare and exophthalmos are likely due to Grave's disease.

B. The sensitivity of bulging flanks for ascites is very low.

C. Pooled studies of the physical examination for ascites show that bulging flanks have a sensitivity of 81% and a specificity of 59% for the presence of ascites.

D. His clinical history and physical appearance are most consistent with left-sided heart failure.

Answer: C

The pooled sensitivity of bulging flanks for the presence of ascites is 81% and the specificity is 59%. This patient's history of congenital heart disease and symptoms (lower extremity edema and increasing abdominal girth) are consistent with right-sided heart failure. His stare and exophthalmos are due to markedly increased venous pressure from high right heart pressures and resultant high jugular venous pressure. The retro-orbital and venous plexus of the eyes drains into the cavernous sinus and jugular venous systems. The stare and exophthalmos of right heart failure can be reversed with treatment of congestive heart failure.

EARNEST DL, HURST JW. Exophthalmos, stare, increase in intraocular pressure and systolic propulsion of the eyeballs due to congestive heart failure. *Am J Cardiol* 1970;26:351–354.

WILLIAMS JW, SIMEL DL. The rational clinical examination: does this patient have ascites? *JAMA* 1992;19:2645–2648.

Case 27

Images contributed by Mona Litvak

An 81-year-old woman is admitted from the Emergency Department (ED) to your service for a fever of 40°C, chills, confusion, and right flank pain. She has a history of poorly controlled diabetes mellitus, recurrent urinary tract infections, chronic kidney disease, and renal staghorn calculi. On physical examination she has mild right midabdominal pain and marked right costovertebral angle tenderness. Her white blood cell count is 11,900/mm^3 and her urinalysis is remarkable for 2+ leukocyte esterase and nitrites and 110 white blood cells per high power field. The ED physician has obtained a kidney, ureter, and bladder (KUB) radiograph (Fig. 27.1) and the intern subsequently ordered a computed tomographic (CT) scan of the abdomen (Figs. 27.2 and 27.3).

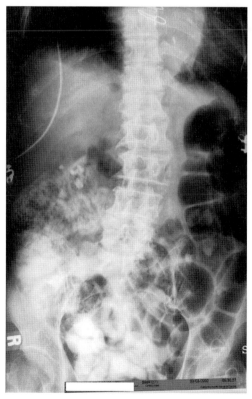

Figure 27.1 KUB radiograph.

Hospital Images: A Clinical Atlas, First Edition. Edited by Paul B. Aronowitz.
© 2012 Wiley-Blackwell. Published 2012 by John Wiley & Sons, Inc.

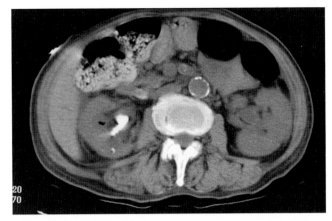

Figure 27.2 CT scan of abdomen.

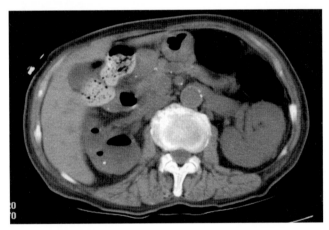

Figure 27.3 CT scan of abdomen.

Question

What is the best subsequent step in this patient's management?

    A. Begin antibiotics and observe.

    B. Begin antibiotics and contact interventional radiology.

    C. Begin antibiotics and contact a urologist for consideration of nephrectomy.

    D. Contact a surgeon for an appendectomy.

Answer: C

This patient has a relatively rare but life-threatening condition known as emphysematous pyelonephritis. Emphysematous pyelonephritis is a severe, necrotizing infection that may result in the presence of gas in the renal parenchyma, collecting system, and perinephric space. The KUB (Fig. 27.4) shows gas within and around her kidney as well as calcifications consistent with staghorn calculi. The CT scans (Figs. 27.5 and 27.6) also show gas within her kidney and the collecting system as well as an area of necrosis.

Emphysematous pyelonephritis, though rare, tends mostly to occur in diabetics, is more common in women, and is also associated with obstruction from nephrolithiasis. While it is possible to manage this disorder with antibiotics and percutaneous drainage, this patient has extensive disease with a large staghorn calculus and areas of renal necrosis. One retrospective study of 48 patients with emphysematous pyelonephritis found an overall mortality rate of 19% but an overall treatment success rate of 90% (9 of 10 patients) with nephrectomy. A meta-analysis of 7 study cohorts, representing 175 patients with emphysematous pyelonephritis, found an overall mortality rate of 25% but ranged from 11% to 42%.

The most common causative bacteria are *Escherichia coli* and *Klebsiella*. This patient's blood and urine grew *E. coli*. She refused surgery or percutaneous drainage for 1 week but continued to have high fevers and pain. She finally agreed to a nephrectomy and recovered without further difficulties after the surgery.

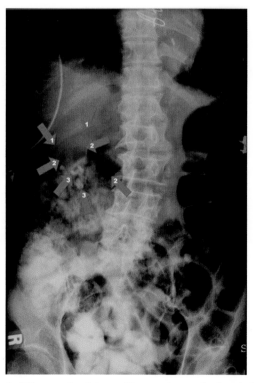

Figure 27.4   Abdominal X-ray; perinephric gas (1), several gas collections in the mid and upper pole (2) of the right kidney suggestive of emphysematous pyelonephritis, and numerous calcifications (3) within the same kidney.

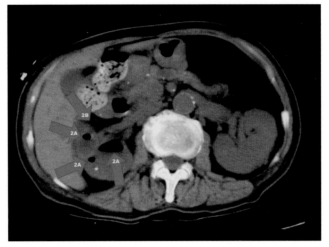

Figure 27.5 Abdominal CT; several gas collections within the right kidney (2A) with necrosis in the upper pole (2B).

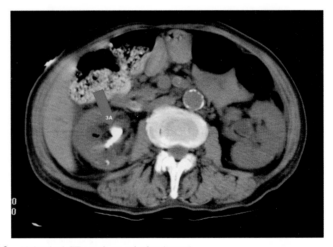

Figure 27.6 Abdominal CT; staghorn calculus (arrow).

FALAGAS ME, et al. Risk factors for mortality in patients with emphysematous pyelonephritis: a meta-analysis. *J Urol* 2007;178;880–885.

HUANG JJ, TSENG CC. Emphysematous pyelonephritis: clinicoradiological classification, management, prognosis, and pathogenesis. *Arch Intern Med* 2000;160:797–805.

Case 28

You are called to see a patient for admission from the Emergency Department (ED) who presents with complaints of fever, chills, and facial redness (Fig. 28.1) and pain.

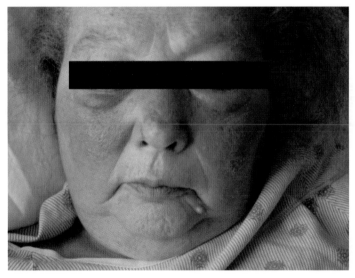

Figure 28.1

Hospital Images: A Clinical Atlas, First Edition. Edited by Paul B. Aronowitz.
© 2012 Wiley-Blackwell. Published 2012 by John Wiley & Sons, Inc.

Question 1

What would the most appropriate next step be in the management of this patient?

A. Admit for high-dose steroids, cytoxan, and urgent rheumatology consultation.

B. Add anti-nuclear antibodies to her laboratory tests and politely explain to the ED doctor that she can be discharged with follow-up with her primary care doctor in 24 hours.

C. Order an anti-Jo1 antibody test, begin prednisone, and admit to the hospital.

D. Admit to the hospital, order blood cultures, and begin intravenous antibiotics to cover for *Streptococcus pyogenes* and *Staphylococcus aureus*.

E. Discharge home on oral antibiotics with close follow-up by her primary care physician.

Question 2

Which of the following best describes the condition illustrated in Figure 28.1?

A. It involves the fascia.

B. It involves the deep dermis and subcutaneous fat tissues.

C. It involves the upper dermis.

D. It is confined to the epidermis.

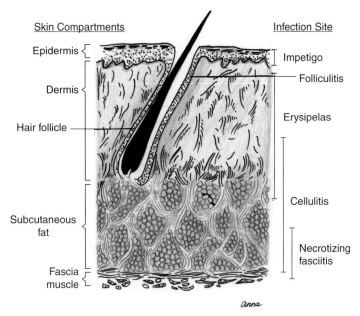

Figure 28.2

Answer 1: D

This patient had a fairly abrupt onset of a superficial cellulitis consistent with erysipelas. Erysipelas may be preceded by a prodrome of flulike illness that occurs hours to days prior to the appearance of the erythema. Though the treatment is essentially the same, several features distinguish erysipelas from cellulitis. In erysipelas the borders tend to be well delineated, as in this patient, in contrast to cellulitis—where it is frequently difficult to distinguish where the rash begins and ends. Another classic feature of erysipelas illustrated in this patient is the *peau d'orange* (orange-skin-like) appearance overlying involved skin. Erysipelas usually occurs on the lower extremities (75–90%) but occurs on the face in 3–10% of cases. It is usually caused by *Streptococcus pyogenes*, but other causative organisms include other beta-hemolytic streptococci, *Staphylococcus aureus*, and enterococci. Gram-negative organisms are a rare cause of erysipelas.

Patients with erysipelas do not necessarily need admission to the hospital but, because of the extent of facial involvement in this patient and her age, hospitalization is reasonable. Though drawing blood cultures is a standard next step, they are only positive in 5–10% of patients with erysipelas.

The facial rash of systemic lupus erythematosus tends to spare the nasolabial folds; this patient has a rash that involves the nasolabial folds, making lupus much less likely. Sunlight exposure tends to trigger the malar rash of lupus and the angle at which light strikes the face tends to spare the nasolabial folds, which are slightly shaded. She also lacks other clinical history suggestive of lupus other than fever and malar rash.

Answer 2: C

Impetigo is a superficial infection involving the epidermis. Erysipelas is an infection of the upper dermis. Cellulitis involves the deeper dermis and subcutaneous fat. Necrotizing fasciitis involves the fascia with relative sparing of the overlying skin and underlying muscle, thus frequently making it a difficult entity to promptly recognize. (See Fig. 28.2.)

Notably, this patient has a small area of "honey crusting" at the left midcheek, which could easily have provided a portal of entry for the causative bacterium.

LOPEZ FA, LARTCHENKO S. Skin and soft tissue infections. *Infect Dis Clin North Am* 2006; 20:759–772.

O'CONNOR K, PAAUW D. Erysipelas: rare but important cause of malar rash. *Am J Med* 2010; 123(5):414–416.

SWARTZ MN. Cellulitis. *N Engl J Med* 2004;350:904–912.

Case 29

You are asked to perform a medical consultation in the Emergency Department. The patient is a 29-year-old woman who complains of red, tender "bumps" on her shins and ankles. She grew up in Minnesota but has lived in San Francisco for 8 years. She teaches at a local elementary school. She has not travelled in the past year, denies sick contacts, cough, shortness of breath, weight loss, or sweats. She does not take any medications except a daily vitamin. She says that she thinks she may have had a sore throat 2 or 3 weeks ago but that it went away after a couple of days. The lesions are bilateral (Figs. 29.1 and 29.2), erythematous, tender, and not fluctuant and they are confined to the extensor surfaces of her lower legs and ankles. The rest of her physical examination and vital signs are normal.

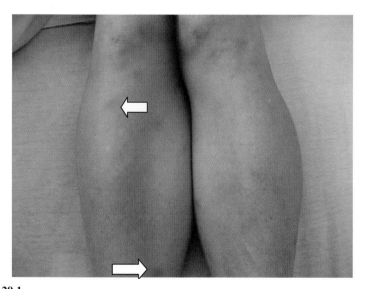

Figure 29.1

Hospital Images: A Clinical Atlas, First Edition. Edited by Paul B. Aronowitz.
© 2012 Wiley-Blackwell. Published 2012 by John Wiley & Sons, Inc.

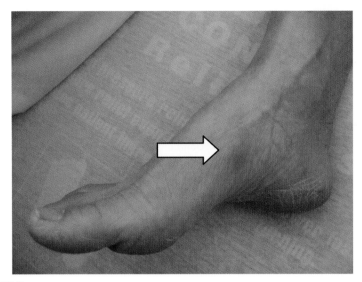

Figure 29.2

Question 1

What advice regarding the next steps in the care of this patient would you provide to the ED physician?

A. Obtain a chest X-ray and begin a short course of corticosteroids if it is normal.

B. Place a PPD skin test, obtain a chest X-ray, and test for the presence of anti-streptolysin O antibodies.

C. Consult Gastroenterology for colonoscopy and upper endoscopy with duodenal biopsy.

D. Start the patient on nonsteroidal anti-inflammatory drugs (NSAIDs) and reassure her that these lesions will resolve in 3–6 weeks.

Question 2

If you were to obtain a biopsy of these lesions, histopathology would likely reveal:

A. Clusters of multinucleated giant cells

B. Nonspecific hemorrhage into subcutaneous tissue

C. Septal panniculitis

D. Leukocytoclastic vasculitis

Answer 1: B

These lesions are erythema nodosum. They usually occur on the anterior aspects of the lower extremities and ankles but may occur on the extensor surfaces of the upper extremities and trunk. In adults these lesions are much more common in women, but in children the male-to-female ratio is 1:1. The mean age of presentation in adults is 20–30 years. While the majority of erythema nodosum are idiopathic, important associated diseases include sarcoidosis, streptococcal infections (especially beta-hemolytic streptococcus), tuberculosis, inflammatory bowel disease (IBD), fungal infections, and drugs. A thorough history and physical examination and consideration of local disease patterns should guide the subsequent evaluation. Placement of a PPD skin test, a chest X-ray, and anti–streptolysin O antibodies are all reasonable tests in this patient. The chest X-ray will help rule out active pulmonary tuberculosis or hilar adenopathy characteristic of sarcoidosis. Since streptococcal infections are a common cause of erythema nodosum and the patient is a school teacher who reports having had a sore throat 2 or 3 weeks ago, anti–streptolysin O antibodies could also be helpful in identifying an etiology.

Corticosteroids are usually not indicated for treatment as this is usually a self-limited process. NSAIDs should be the first line of treatment, particularly given that these lesions can be quite painful. Although IBD can be associated with erythema nodosum, this patient does not have any gastrointestinal symptoms, making IBD improbable.

After turning a deep, purplish color, these lesions usually resolve in 3–6 weeks, rarely recur, and never cause ulceration or other significant cosmetic repercussions.

Answer 2: C

Biopsy of erythema nodosum will usually reveal a septal panniculitis—the septum surrounding subcutaneous fat becomes thickened and infiltrated with inflammatory cells. There is no vasculitis associated with this disorder. It is unclear what initiates the septal panniculitis of erythema nodosum, but erythema nodosum is considered to be a hypersensitivity response. It appears that these lesions result from the formation of immune complexes and their deposition within the connective tissue septum that surrounds subcutaneous fat.

REQUENA L, REQUENA C. Erythema nodosum. *Dermatol Online J* 2002;8(1):E4.
SCHWARTZ RA, NERVI SJ. Erythema nodosum: a sign of systemic disease. *Am Acad Fam Phys* 2007;75(5):695–700.

Case 30

Images contributed by David Z. Rose

A 60-year-old man with a long history of tobacco use is brought to the Emergency Department (ED) by his wife due to erratic behavior and a large, painless forehead mass (Figs. 30.1 and 30.2). The patient is admitted to your service for evaluation. You meet the patient's wife in the ED. She says she is worried he has cancer since he was exposed to Agent Orange during his military service in Vietnam. She wants to know your opinion as well as what type of cancer would present "in this extreme way."

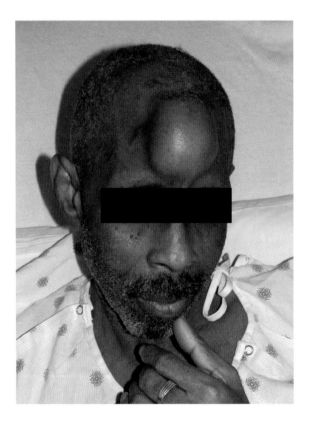

Figure 30.1

Hospital Images: A Clinical Atlas, First Edition. Edited by Paul B. Aronowitz.
© 2012 Wiley-Blackwell. Published 2012 by John Wiley & Sons, Inc.

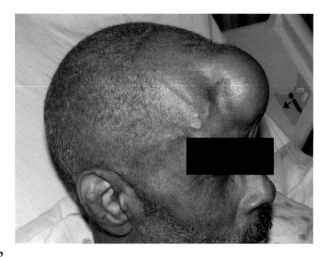

Figure 30.2

Question 1

Which of the following would you tell her?

   A. This could be a primary sarcoma of the skull from Agent Orange exposure.

   B. This is most likely a metastatic skull lesion from a tobacco-related cancer.

   C. This is likely a metastatic skull lesion from thyroid carcinoma.

   D. This is likely to be a metastatic skull lesion from prostate cancer related to Agent Orange exposure.

A computed tomographic (CT) scan of the chest reveals an 8 × 8-cm mass in the right lower lobe that is encasing the pulmonary artery. Biopsy of the forehead mass reveals squamous cell carcinoma. A CT scan of the head (Fig. 30.3) reveals a large mass extending from the frontal bone intracranially with displacement of both frontal lobes. The patient's cousin, a physical therapist in another state, pages you and asks you what stage this patient's lung cancer is.

Question 2

Which of the following would you tell him it is?

   A. Stage IIA

   B. Stage IIIA

   C. Stage IIIB

   D. Stage IV

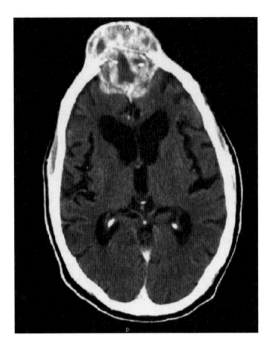

Figure 30.3

Answer 1: B

The patient's long history of tobacco use is most germane to this patient's illness. You would explain to the patient's wife that, although further studies and a biopsy of the mass or other accessible tissue need to be done before you can be certain, you think it much less likely that Agent Orange exposure has played a role in this patient's forehead mass.

Studies of veterans who were exposed to Agent Orange are still somewhat unclear regarding increased cancer risk, though some studies have indicated that these veterans are at increased risk of prostate cancer. Prostate cancer can metastasize to the skull, though breast cancer and lung cancer are more common culprits for this type of presentation. Skeletal metastatic disease as the primary presentation of lung cancer only occurs in 2% of patients with lung cancer. Besides breast, lung, and prostate, other cancers that can metastasize to the skull include thyroid cancer, melanoma, and multiple myeloma.

Answer 2: D

Regardless of tumor (T) or lymph nodes (N), this patient has distant metastatic (M) disease—M1; M1 with any T or N is Stage IV. This patient continued to be confused and, at the request of his wife, was subsequently discharged home under hospice care. He died 2 weeks later.

SILVESTRI GA, et al. Noninvasive staging of non-small cell lung cancer: ACCP evidence-based clinical practice guidelines. *Chest* 2007;132(3 Suppl):178S–201S.
ROSE DZ, et al. Extreme presentation of bony metastatic disease. *J Hosp Med* 2007;2(2):110–111.
SHAH SR, TERRIS MK. Agent Orange exposure, Vietnam War veterans, and the risk of prostate cancer. *Cancer* 2008;113(9):2382–2384.

Case 31

Image contributed by Alissa Detz

A 41-year-old woman is admitted from the Emergency Department to your "nocturnist" service at 2 AM for complaints of 1 month of increasing fatigue, dyspnea on exertion, gingival tenderness, and hyperplasia (Fig. 31.1). Her complete blood count reveals a platelet count of 32,000 cells per microliter, white blood cell count 16,000 cells per microliter, and hemoglobin 6.4 g/dL. You review her peripheral smear, which reveals a paucity of platelets, normochromic and normocytic anemia, and occasional blast cells.

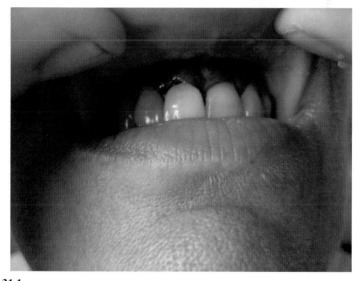

Figure 31.1

Hospital Images: A Clinical Atlas, First Edition. Edited by Paul B. Aronowitz.
© 2012 Wiley-Blackwell. Published 2012 by John Wiley & Sons, Inc.

Question

This presentation is *most* consistent with which of the following:

    A. Chronic lymphocytic leukemia (CLL)

    B. Chronic myelogenous leukemia (CML)

    C. Acute promyelocytic leukemia (FAB classification, M3)

    D. Acute monocytic leukemia (FAB classification, M5)

Answer:D

Gingival overgrowth from gingival leukemic infiltrates occurs in approximately 4% of acute myeloid leukemia (AML) patients. However, it is a much more frequent complication of acute monocytic leukemia (M5 FAB classification), occurring in 67% of cases, than of acute myelomonocytic leukemia (M4), occurring in 19% of cases. It is uncommon in chronic forms of leukemia, and in one large retrospective study of 1076 patients with leukemia it did not occur in any patients with CLL or CML. The exception to this was CML in blastic phase, where 3% of patients had gingival hyperplasia.

Although common in both M4 and M5 AML, this is a poorly understood complication of leukemia. Infiltrated gingiva is usually swollen, glazed, spongy in consistency, and devoid of stippling, and its color is bright red to purple. Biopsy, though usually not necessary, shows leukemic cell infiltration. Though dental caries and poor dental hygiene are thought to put these patients at higher risk of infectious complications, it does not appear to increase the likelihood of gingival infiltration. Of note, edentulous patients with AML do not develop this complication—also a poorly understood aspect of this disease. It has been hypothesized that local irritation and trauma (in the presence of teeth) leads to the presence of gingival infiltration. Gingival hyperplasia from AML reverses with response to chemotherapy.

COOPER CL, LOEWEN R, SHORE T. Gingival hyperplasia complicating acute myelomonocytic leukemia. *J Can Dent Assoc* 2000;66:78–79.

DEMIRER S, et al. Gingival hyperplasia as an early diagnostic oral manifestation in acute monocytic leukemia: a case report. *European J Dent* 2007;1:111–114.

DREIZEN S, et al. Malignant gingival and skin "infiltrates" in adult leukemia. *Oral Surg Oral Med Oral Pathol* 1983;55:572–579.

Case 32

Image contributed by Julie Chen and Sharon Chinthrajah

You are consulted by the Emergency Department (ED) physician about a 56-year-old man with a past history of arthritis with severe pain in his right knee and left metatarsal phalangeal joint. The patient has a history of multiple kidney stones over the past 10 years. His serum creatinine is 1.8 mg/dL and uric acid is 12.6 mg/dL. His hands are abnormal (Fig. 32.1) and his right knee and the base of his left great toe are warm, swollen, and exquisitely tender.

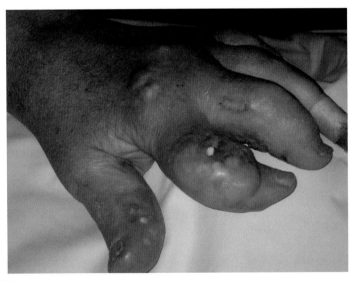

Figure 32.1

Hospital Images: A Clinical Atlas, First Edition. Edited by Paul B. Aronowitz.
© 2012 Wiley-Blackwell. Published 2012 by John Wiley & Sons, Inc.

Question

How would you advise the ED physician to manage this patient's knee and foot pain?

    A. Discharge the patient with strict instructions for bed rest and to follow up with you in 1 week.

    B. Administer 1 dose of intravenous ketorolac in the ED and discharge the patient with a 1-week course of ibuprofen.

    C. Administer 2 g of colchicine intravenously over 1 hour.

    D. Discharge the patient with colchicine 0.6 mg orally every 2 hours until symptoms improve or diarrhea and/or vomiting occur.

    E. Administer 100 mg of methylprednisolone and then discharge the patient on 60 mg of oral prednisone per day with a tapering dose over 10 days.

Answer:E

Although an acute gout flare will gradually resolve over several days, the numerous options for treatment and rapid improvement of gout make bed rest a less optimal choice. Ketorolac has an onset of action of 30–45 minutes, and a patient with acute gout can attain rapid improvement in the ED. However, ketorolac and ibuprofen are nonsteroidal anti-inflammatory drugs (NSAIDs) and therefore are poor choices given this patient's chronic kidney disease. Intravenous colchicine is not used to treat acute gout anymore given its potential to cause venous sclerosis and bone marrow toxicity.

Although oral colchicine is not an unreasonable choice for acute gout, the rather primitive aspects of treating a patient until side effects occur has made colchicine a less favored choice. Intravenous methylprednisolone will achieve rapid therapeutic effect and a short, tapering course of prednisone has a relatively low risk-to-benefit profile. An additional option not presented here would be to inject the knee and the toe with intra-articular corticosteroids.

CHEN J, CHINTHRAJAH RS, ARONOWITZ PB. Severe tophaceous gout. *J Hosp Med* 2007;2(3):194.

KEITH MP, GILLILAND WR. Updates in the management of gout. *Am J Med* 2007;120(3):221–224.

NUKI G. Treatment of crystal arthropathy—history and advances. *Rheum Dis Clin North Am* 2006; 32:333–357.

TERKELTAUB RA. Gout. *N Engl J Med* 2003;349(17):1647–1655.

Case 33

Image contributed by Marina Trilleskaya

A 56-year-old man undergoes a four-vessel coronary bypass procedure. Five days after surgery you are contacted by his nurse because he developed the sudden onset of pleuritic chest pain and mild shortness of breath. On physical examination his blood pressure is at baseline, his heart rate is 102 beats per minute, his oxygen saturation is 91% on room air, and he is afebrile. Except for tachycardia, an electrocardiogram (EKG) is unchanged compared with his pre-operative EKG. His chest radiograph is shown in Figure 33.1.

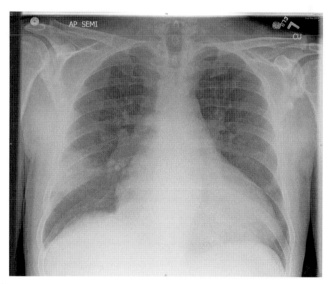

Figure 33.1

Hospital Images: A Clinical Atlas, First Edition. Edited by Paul B. Aronowitz.
© 2012 Wiley-Blackwell. Published 2012 by John Wiley & Sons, Inc.

Question 1

What is the best subsequent step in this patient's management?

   A. Order blood cultures and sputum Gram stain and cultures, and begin intravenous antibiotics.

   B. Contact the patient's cardiothoracic surgeon for urgent pericardiocentesis.

   C. Begin heparin and obtain a pulmonary computed tomographic (CT) angiogram as soon as possible.

   D. Administer 20 mg furosemide via intravenous route and observe for improvement.

Question 2

Regarding this patient's acute medical disorder, which of the following is the most common finding on chest radiographs?

   A. Atelectasis

   B. Pleural effusion

   C. Bilateral pulmonary vascular redistribution

   D. Elevated hemidiaphragm

   E. Dilated pulmonary artery

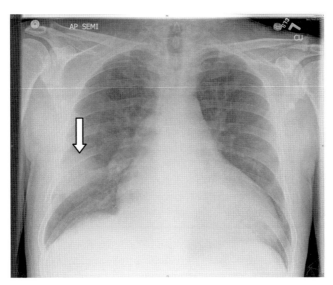

Figure 33.2

Answer 1: C

This chest radiograph shows Hampton's hump, a wedge-shaped area of pleural infarction from pulmonary embolism (Fig. 33.2, arrow). Hampton's hump is an uncommon finding in pulmonary embolism, seen in less than 10% of patients with this disorder. Other *uncommon* findings include Westermark's sign (focal decreased vascularity) and Palla's sign (dilated descending right pulmonary artery).

Answer 2: C

The chest radiograph in pulmonary embolism is frequently abnormal and may show atelectasis (most common finding), elevated hemidiaphragm, small pleural effusion(s), and, rarely, dilated pulmonary artery or arteries. These findings are nonspecific. Pulmonary vascular redistribution would be consistent with volume overload states but would not be expected to occur in the setting of an acute pulmonary embolism. The chest X-ray is not a good test for cinching the diagnosis of pulmonary embolism, but it is a good place to start to rule out other acute processes that may explain a patient's symptoms. This patient's CT angiogram showed multiple pulmonary emboli and he was treated accordingly.

AKPINA MG, GOODMAN LR. Imaging of pulmonary thromboembolism. *Clin Chest Med* 2008;29: 107–116

WORSLEY DF, et al. Chest radiographic findings in patients with acute pulmonary embolism: observations from the PIOPED Study. *Radiology* 1993;189:133–136.

Case 34

Image contributed by Alireza Ghotb

An 86-year-old Russian immigrant with coronary artery disease and hypertension is admitted to the hospital for left-sided chest pain radiating to his back for the past 2 days. His discomfort started as a bandlike sensation in his mid to lower left chest wall. He also described the pain to be "like lying on top of wrinkled sheets." On the morning of presentation the patient experienced worsening of pain in the same area, accompanied by a burning sensation, and he came to the Emergency Department (ED). At that time his skin examination was normal and he was found to have an unchanged electrocardiogram without acute changes, normal laboratory studies, including blood urea nitrogen (BUN), creatinine, troponin I, and creatine kinase, and a normal chest X-ray. A computed tomographic (CT) scan of the chest to rule out aortic dissection or pulmonary embolus was performed in the ED, and it was negative. The following morning as you are assessing him he complains about a new rash on his back and chest (Figs. 34.1 and 34.2).

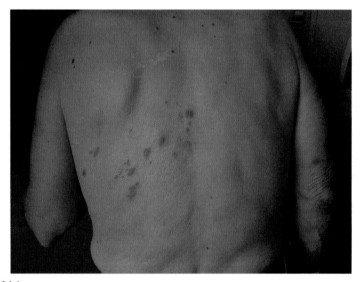

Figure 34.1

Hospital Images: A Clinical Atlas, First Edition. Edited by Paul B. Aronowitz.
© 2012 Wiley-Blackwell. Published 2012 by John Wiley & Sons, Inc.

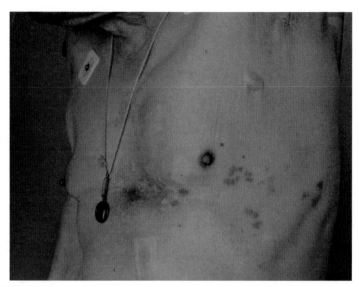

Figure 34.2

Question 1

Which of the following is *not* a potential complication of this patient's disorder?

   A. Encephalitis

   B. A pain syndrome lasting for months to years

   C. Distal peripheral neuropathy

   D. Delayed contralateral hemiparesis

   E. Pneumonitis

Question 2

What is the most appropriate next step in this patient's care?

   A. Viral and bacterial culture of skin lesions

   B. Initiation of antiviral therapy, placement of sterile, nonocclusive, nonadherent dressing over the skin lesions, and discharge home

   C. Nonurgent evaluation for underlying HIV infection or cancer

   D. Placement of sterile, nonocclusive, nonadherent dressing over skin lesions and discharge home

Just prior to discharge the nursing staff pages you at the request of the patient's wife. She was a physician in Russia and has several questions about the patient's treatment and prognosis. She is concerned about side effects of the antiviral medication you started the patient on and wants to know if it is safe, whether it will speed healing, and whether it will decrease complications of his condition.

Question 3

Which of the following would you tell her?

A. The antiviral medication has a good safety profile, will halt the formation of new lesions more quickly, and will accelerate the rate of healing compared with not giving the medication, but it will not decrease his chance of developing postherpetic neuralgia.

B. The antiviral medication has a good safety profile and will not affect healing or new lesion formation, but it will markedly decrease his chance of developing postherpetic neuralgia.

C. The antiviral medication has a good safety profile, will halt the formation of new lesions more quickly, will accelerate the rate of healing, and will also significantly decrease the duration of pain from postherpetic neuralgia compared with not giving the medication.

D. The antiviral medication is very safe in the setting of the patient's normal renal function but there is little definitive evidence about its efficacy.

Herpes zoster, also known as shingles, occurs from the reactivation of latent varicella-zoster virus (VZV) within the sensory ganglia from prior chicken pox infection. It commonly presents as painful unilateral vesicular eruption that occurs in one dermatome. The rash of herpes zoster classically starts as erythematous papules that quickly evolve into clusters of vesicles; the thoracic and lumbar dermatomes are most commonly involved.

Approximately 75% of patients will have prodromal pain in the dermatome where the rash subsequently appears. The pain often precedes the rash by days but the time can be as long as weeks. It is often described as a burning or stabbing sensation and can be quite severe, sometimes prompting workup for alternate diagnoses such as acute coronary syndrome, aortic dissection, and cholecystitis.

Answer 1: C

Encephalitis, postherpetic neuralgia, a syndrome of delayed contralateral hemiparesis, and pneumonitis are all potential complications of herpes zoster. Distal peripheral neuropathy is not a complication of herpes zoster. Other possible complications include disseminated zoster, Bell's palsy, myelitis, secondary cutaneous bacterial infections, retinal necrosis, and postherpetic itch as well as anxiety and depression related to the disabling effects of postherpetic neuralgia.

Answer 2: B

In the early stages of herpes zoster, antiviral therapy has been shown to be beneficial. Good skin care, including nonocclusive, nonadherent sterile dressing to decrease friction with clothing, is also recommended. When the diagnosis of herpes zoster is fairly obvious, it is not necessary to perform cultures or other testing. Increasing age is an important risk factor for developing herpes zoster. The lifetime risk of this disease is approximately 10–20%. Though patients with neoplastic diseases are at increased risk of developing herpes zoster, it is not currently recommended that patients presenting with zoster undergo evaluation for underlying malignancy. However, in patients younger than age 50 presenting with herpes zoster, human immunodeficiency virus (HIV) testing should be considered. The incidence of herpes zoster is 29 cases per 1000 person-years in HIV-positive persons in contrast to 2 cases per 1000 person-years in HIV-negative persons.

Answer 3: C

Though topical antiviral therapy is not efficacious or recommended, systemic antiviral therapy is recommended based on various clinical trials and meta-analyses. Acyclovir, famciclovir, and valacyclovir are all remarkably safe agents (though they should be dose adjusted in the setting of renal failure). These agents are phosphorylated by viral thymidine kinase to a triphosphate form that inhibits viral replication.

Most trials of these agents were done in patients presenting within 72 hours of the onset of rash, but their use should still be considered in patients presenting more than 72 hours after onset of rash given their low risk and potential benefit. The usual duration of treatment is 7 days. The data to support use of any of these three agents is well established, and valacyclovir and famciclovir tend to be preferred over acyclovir due to simpler dosing regimens and better pharmacokinetics. These drugs have been shown to shorten the duration of viral shedding, diminish the formation of new vesicles more quickly, and accelerate healing while also decreasing acute pain and duration of postherpetic neuralgia.

Oral corticosteroids remain controversial in the treatment of herpes zoster to the point where they should probably not be initiated in patients with diabetes, hypertension, or peptic ulcer disease.

DWORKIN RH, et al. Recommendations for the management of herpes zoster. *Clin Infect Dis* 2007;44 (Suppl 1):S1-S26.

GNANN JW, WHITLEY RJ. Herpes zoster. *N Engl J Med* 2002;347(5):340–346.

YAWN BP, et al. A population-based study of the incidence and complication rates of herpes zoster before zoster vaccine introduction. *Mayo Clin Proc* 2007;82(11):1341–1349.

Case 35

Images contributed by Ryan Wong

A 62-year-old woman with a history of Munchausen's syndrome presents with complaints of 2 days of progressive weakness. She reports ingesting a large number of potassium chloride tablets. Potassium level on a stat chemistry panel is 10.4 mmol/L, and her initial electrocardiogram (EKG) is shown in Figure 35.1. Her blood tests reveal normal blood urea nitrogen (BUN) and serum creatinine levels.

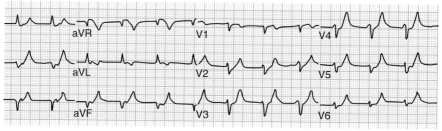

Figure 35.1

Hospital Images: A Clinical Atlas, First Edition. Edited by Paul B. Aronowitz.
© 2012 Wiley-Blackwell. Published 2012 by John Wiley & Sons, Inc.

Question 1

Which of the following is the most rapid-acting initial therapy for this patient?

    A. 50 g of intravenous dextrose followed immediately by 10 units of intravenous insulin

    B. Albuterol 0.5 mL in 2.5 mL saline administered via nebulizer

    C. 30 g polystyrene sodium sulfonate sorbitol liquid (Kayexylate) by mouth

    D. 1 ampule (50 mEq) of sodium bicarbonate intravenously

    E. 1 ampule (1 g) calcium gluconate intravenously

Figure 35.2 shows an EKG shortly after administration of calcium gluconate, sodium bicarbonate, and dextrose with insulin therapy. A repeat potassium level returns at 9.2 mmol/L.

Question 2

At this juncture, what is the best subsequent management step?

    A. Repeat previous therapies and obtain emergent nephrology consultation for dialysis.

    B. Administer Kayexylate and wait at least 2 hours before repeating a serum potassium level.

    C. Assume that the potassium level is a laboratory error and repeat it.

    D. Perform an emergent computer tomographic (CT) scan of the chest, abdomen, and pelvis to evaluate for lymphoma with spontaneous tumor lysis syndrome.

Question 3

Regarding electrocardiographic changes due to hyperkalemia, which statement is most accurate?

    A. EKG changes cannot be relied upon to exclude life-threatening hyperkalemia.

    B. EKG changes are both sensitive and specific for predicting cardiac arrest from hyperkalemia.

    C. EKG changes always progress from peaked T waves to wide QRS complex to "sine wave" pattern prior to cardiac arrest.

    D. A potassium level should always be checked in the setting of EKG changes thought to be due to hyperkalemia prior to initiating therapy to lower potassium.

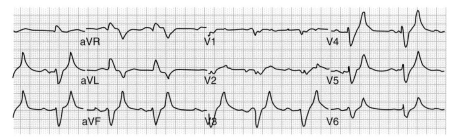

Figure 35.2

Answer 1: E

This patient has a history consistent with a potassium overdose, an unusual cause of hyperkalemia in a patient with otherwise normal renal function. Her initial EKG shows peaked T waves, widening of the QRS complex, and loss of P waves. All of the listed options are reasonable therapies to help lower potassium in the urgent setting. Calcium gluconate stabilizes myocardial cells by directly antagonizing the membrane effects of potassium and works in 2–3 minutes. Sodium bicarbonate alkalinizes the extracellular space, causing hydrogen ions to be released as a buffer in exchange for potassium; this effect begins within 5–10 minutes of administration. Albuterol (a beta-2-agonist) given via nebulizer acts to lower potassium in 30–90 minutes and works by driving potassium into cells by increasing Na-K-ATPase activity. Insulin drives potassium into cells by enhancing Na-K-ATPase activity in skeletal muscle and should be given with glucose to avoid hypoglycemia. Dextrose–insulin therapy takes approximately 15 minutes to take effect, with peak action approximately 60 minutes after administration. Of note, each of these therapies is capable of reducing serum potassium by 0.5–1.5 meq/L, though these effects may only be transient.

Answer 2: A

The three steps of treating hyperkalemia include (1) antagonizing the effects of hyperkalemia, (2) emergent reduction of potassium levels by driving potassium into cells, and (3) removal of potassium from the body. Even with aggressive action, this patient would require dialysis, as demonstrated by her repeat electrocardiogram showing peaked T waves and marked widening of the QRS complex. In the setting of a markedly elevated serum potassium and the EKG abnormalities seen in Figure 35.2, it would be dangerous to delay immediate, aggressive potassium lowering while repeating the serum potassium level or waiting for Kayexylate to work.

Answer 3: A

Electrocardiographic changes are not always a reliable marker of hyperkalemia. Hyperkalemia greater than 6.5 mmol/L should be treated aggressively regardless of the absence of EKG changes. There is little medical literature examining sensitivity and specificity of EKG changes in the setting of hyperkalemia, and the EKG, while useful, should not be the main determinant of the decision to lower potassium levels urgently or emergently.

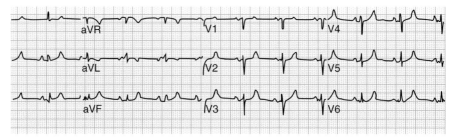

Figure 35.3 Patient's postdialysis EKG.

Case 36

While you are busy evaluating the fifth admission of your nocturnal hospitalist shift, the Emergency Department (ED) physician asks you to "take a quick look" at the fingernails of a 57-year-old man (Figs. 36.1 and 36.2) with a long history of Barrett's esophagus and several months of progressive dysphagia. The patient has come to the ED for complaints of profound fatigue and dyspnea on exertion.

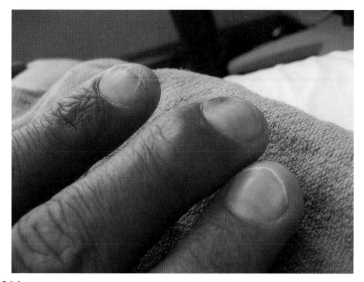

Figure 36.1

Hospital Images: A Clinical Atlas, First Edition. Edited by Paul B. Aronowitz.
© 2012 Wiley-Blackwell. Published 2012 by John Wiley & Sons, Inc.

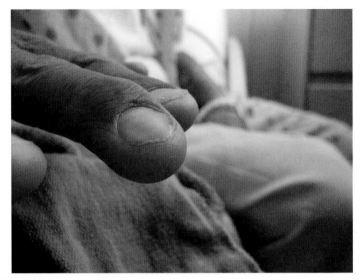

Figure 36.2

Question

What abnormality would you expect to find when his ED evaluation is complete?

    A. Proteinuria

    B. Hematuria

    C. A right upper lobe lung mass on his chest radiograph

    D. Anemia

Answer: D

This patient has koilonychia, otherwise known as spooning of the nails. A transverse and longitudinal concavity of the nail occurs, causing the nail to look spoon-shaped. Koilonychia is generally associated with chronic iron-deficiency anemia but can also be familial, idiopathic, or related to sulfur–protein deficiency, hyperthyroidism, or hemochromatosis. The pathogenesis of koilonychia is not known, but the condition is reversible when iron is repleted and anemia is corrected.

This patient's evaluation revealed a microcytic anemia with a hemoglobin of 6.5 g/dL, iron deficiency, and a severe esophageal stricture with severe gastritis and esophagitis. He did not have cancer.

HARRISON S, BERGFELD WF. Diseases of the hair and nails. *Med Clin North Am* 2009;93:1195–1209.
KUMAR G, et al. Images in emergency medicine: koilonychia. *Ann Emerg Med* 2007;49(2);243–244.

Case 37

Written by Alissa Detz

An 86-year-old previously healthy Ukrainian immigrant presents with 1 month of rash on his torso and extremities. There is no associated pain or pruritis. Review of systems reveals a history of slight fatigue but he denies fevers, chills, weight change, sick contacts, or recent travel.

Physical examination reveals multiple papules, which are symmetrically distributed on his torso (Figs. 37.1 and 37.2) and lower extremities. Laboratory studies reveal thrombocytopenia with a platelet count of 11,000/μL and an elevated white

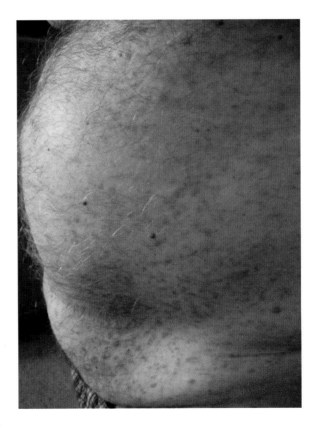

Figure 37.1

Hospital Images: A Clinical Atlas, First Edition. Edited by Paul B. Aronowitz.
© 2012 Wiley-Blackwell. Published 2012 by John Wiley & Sons, Inc.

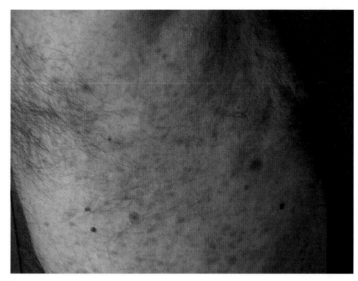

Figure 37.2

blood cell count of 37,000 cells per microliter with numerous blast cells seen on his peripheral smear. A skin biopsy reveals infiltration of the dermis with myeloid cells.

Question 1

What is this patient's diagnosis and most likely associated underlying malignancy?

    A. Sweet's syndrome associated with acute myeloid leukemia (AML)

    B. Leukemia cutis associated with AML

    C. Petechiae associated with chronic myeloid leukemia (CML)

    D. Erythema gyratum repens associated with bronchogenic lung cancer

Question 2

Which of the following statements is true regarding this rash?

    A. It precedes the other manifestations of malignancy in most patients.

    B. It is more common in adults than in children with this malignancy.

    C. It often occurs in areas of previous injury or skin breakdown.

    D. It is the most common skin manifestation of this malignancy.

    E. Presence of this rash predicts a better prognosis.

Answer 1: B

Leukemia cutis is a cutaneous manifestation of leukemia characterized by infiltration of the skin with myeloid or lymphoid leukemic cells. It can occur in a variety of leukemias and myeloproliferative disorders and affects 10–15% of patients diagnosed with acute myeloid leukemia (AML). The rash is typically composed of red-brown or violaceous papules, as seen in this patient. The pathophysiology of leukemia cutis is not well understood, but the leading hypothesis is that expression of chemokine receptors and adhesion molecule receptors causes migration of leukemic cells to the skin. Further evaluation of this patient with bone marrow biopsy revealed more than 20% myeloid blast cells, confirming the diagnosis of AML.

Sweet's syndrome, or acute febrile neutrophilic dermatosis, is another cutaneous manifestation of AML. Sweet's syndrome can occur in individuals with leukemia and myeloproliferative diseases but also may be related to infection, drugs, or immunodeficiency. Individuals with Sweet's syndrome usually present with fever, neutrophilia, and a painful rash. The rash typically consists of red nodules or plaques, and biopsy will reveal neutrophilic infiltrate rather than the myeloid cells seen in this case.

Petechiae are nonblanching lesions 1–2 mm in size and are caused by red blood cells extravasating into the skin. Erythema gyratum repens is a rare paraneoplastic rash that is serpiginous, erythematous, and pruritic. It is most often associated with lung cancer but also can be seen in individuals with esophageal cancer and breast cancer.

Answer 2: C

Leukemia cutis most commonly affects the legs but can also involve the arms, back, scalp, and face. It tends to appear in areas of previous inflammation. The rash can be localized to surgical scars or sites of previous herpes zoster infections, although in this patient it occurred more diffusely. Leukemia cutis most often occurs after systemic leukemia has been diagnosed. This disease only occurs before bone marrow or blood involvement in a minority of individuals (<10%). Leukemia cutis is more common in children, affecting 30% of individuals with congenital leukemia.

A variety of skin findings may be present in individuals with AML. Patients commonly exhibit pallor due to anemia, and petechiae or ecchymoses due to thrombocytopenia. Leukemia cutis only affects 10–15% of AML patients.

The presence of leukemia cutis indicates a poor prognosis and a more aggressive disease course. Most patients with leukemia cutis die within 1 year. However, AML has a poor prognosis in older patients even without leukemia cutis. Only 40–60% of these patients will respond to chemotherapy, and the median survival of older individuals with AML is 7–12 months. This patient died from complications of chemotherapy-related neutropenia and sepsis less than 5 months after his diagnosis.

Buck T, et al. Sweet's syndrome with hematologic disorders: a review and reappraisal. *Int J Derm* 2008;47:775–782.

Cho-Vega HJ, et al. Leukemia cutis. *Am J Pathol* 2008;129:130–142.

Eubanks LE, McBurney E, Reed R. Erythema gyratum repens. *Am J Med Sci* 2001;321(5):302–305.

Lowenberg B, Drowning J, Burnett A. Acute myeloid leukemia. *N Engl J Med* 1999; 344(14):1051–1062.

Case **38**

Image contributed by Michael Chen
Written by Yile Ding

A 52-year-old woman with cirrhosis is admitted to your service with large-volume upper gastrointestinal bleeding from esophageal varices. During resuscitation she receives a large amount of blood products, including 18 units of packed red blood cells, 17 units of fresh frozen plasma, 2 units of cryoprecipitate, and 1 unit of platelets. After the patient is stabilized, an electrocardiogram (EKG; Fig. 38.1) is obtained by an Intensive Care Unit (ICU) nurse because she thinks you would like it done as part of the patient's "routine" admission evaluation.

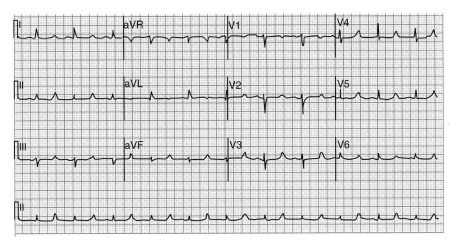

Figure 38.1

Hospital Images: A Clinical Atlas, First Edition. Edited by Paul B. Aronowitz.
© 2012 Wiley-Blackwell. Published 2012 by John Wiley & Sons, Inc.

Question 1

What abnormality is present in this EKG?

- **A.** Atrial fibrillation
- **B.** Prolonged QT interval
- **C.** First-degree atrioventricular block
- **D.** Electrical alternans

Question 2

What would be the best subsequent step in this patient's management?

- **A.** Obtain a prior EKG for comparison and order a serum potassium level.
- **B.** Obtain a prior EKG for comparison and order a serum calcium level.
- **C.** Obtain a prior EKG for comparison, apply cutaneous pacemaker pads, and obtain an urgent cardiology consultation.
- **D.** Obtain a prior EKG for comparison and order a urine toxicology screen.

Question 3

What disorder does this abnormality put this patient at risk of?

- **A.** Complete heart block
- **B.** Cardiac tamponade
- **C.** Torsade de pointes
- **D.** Right atrial enlargement

Answer 1: B

This patient has a long QT interval on the EKG. The QT interval is measured from the beginning of the QRS complex to the end of the T wave; correction is made for heart rate as the QT interval lengthens as heart rate slows and shortens as heart rate increases. Corrected QT (QTc) is most commonly calculated by Bazett's formula: QTc = measured QT interval divided by the square root of the preceding RR interval. In general, a QTc > 450 ms in males or QTc > 460 ms in females is considered abnormal.

Answer 2: B

In this patient's case, the blood product transfusions caused hypocalcemia, which can lead to a prolonged QT interval. The citrate preservative in blood products binds calcium. The patient's QT interval normalized after intravenous calcium repletion.

It would be important to compare her current EKG with her prior to make sure she does not have congenital long QT syndrome. Hypokalemia or hyperkalemia do not cause long QT interval. Until easily reversible disorders, such as hypocalcemia, have been ruled out as an etiology for her long QT interval, pacemaker pads would not be helpful in this setting. A cardiology consultation is not necessary as the QT interval abnormality will reverse quickly with repletion of calcium.

Answer 3: C

Torsades de pointes can develop in the setting of a long QT interval. Long QT can be congenital or acquired in the presence of certain medications or electrolyte abnormalities. A list of drugs associated with a prolonged QT interval is managed online by the Arizona Center for Education and Research on Therapeutics.

MANGAT JS, et al. Hypocalcaemia mimicking long QT syndrome: case report. *Eur J Pediatr* 2008; 167(2):233–235.

RAUTAHARJU PM, et al. AHA/ACCF/HRS recommendations for the standardization and interpretation of the electrocardiogram. *J Am Coll Cardiol* 2009;53(11):982–991.

SIHLER KC, NAPOLITANO LM. Complications of massive transfusion. *Chest* 2010;137(1):209–220.

WOOSLEY RL. Drugs that prolong the QT interval and/or induce torsades de pointes. Tucson (AZ): Arizona Center for Education and Research on Therapeutics. Available at http://www.azcert.org/medical-pros/drug-lists/printable-drug-list.cfm (accessed August 9, 2010)

Case 39

Written by Vanessa London and Nikolas London

A 49-year-old man with a history of morbid obesity and type 2 diabetes mellitus is admitted to your service from the Emergency Department (ED) with a chief complaint of 2 days of epigastric abdominal pain, nausea, and vomiting. By the time you arrive in the ED, the third-year medical student has dilated the patient's eyes and performed a fundoscopic examination (Fig. 39.1).

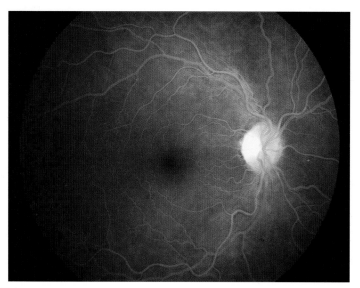

Figure 39.1

Hospital Images: A Clinical Atlas, First Edition. Edited by Paul B. Aronowitz.
© 2012 Wiley-Blackwell. Published 2012 by John Wiley & Sons, Inc.

Question 1

What are the most likely laboratory results for this patient?

A. Total cholesterol, 2306 mg/dL; triglycerides, 22,539 mg/dL; fasting glucose, 160

B. Total cholesterol, 170 mg/dL; triglycerides, 22,539 mg/dL; fasting glucose, 100

C. Total cholesterol, 4500 mg/dL; triglycerides, 854 mg/dL; fasting glucose, 160

D. Total cholesterol, 4500 mg/dL; triglycerides, 854 mg/dL; fasting glucose, 355

Question 2

What is the most likely etiology of this patient's abdominal pain?

A. Pancreatitis

B. Cholecystitis

C. Nonalcoholic steatohepatitis

D. Peptic ulcer disease

Answer 1: A

The creamy, white-pink vessels are diagnostic of lipemia retinalis. This is a rare, underdiagnosed entity seen in the setting of hypertriglyceridemia. This finding is not seen until serum triglyceride level is at least 1000 mg/dL. This patient's cholesterol was 2306 mg/dL and his triglycerides were 22,539 mg/dL as in choice A. Choice B is incorrect because it is very unlikely to have an extremely high triglyceride level with a normal cholesterol level.

Answer 2: D

In the setting of elevated triglycerides, pancreatitis is the most likely etiology of this patient's epigastric abdominal pain. Hypertriglyceridemia causes approximately 7% of acute pancreatitis and is the third most common cause of acute pancreatitis after gallstones and alcohol.

EL-HARAZI SM, KELLAWAY J, ARORA A. Lipaemia retinalis. *Austral N Zealand J Ophthalmol* 1998; 26:255–257.

GAN SI, et al. Hypertriglyceridemia-induced pancreatitis: a case-based review. *World J Gastroenterol* 2006;12(44):7197–7202.

Case 40

Written by Sara Swenson and Andrea Ling
Images contributed by Kjell Jorgenson

A 28-year-old man comes to the Emergency Department (ED) after a syncopal episode. He reports a two-day history of chest pressure, lightheadedness, and dyspnea on exertion. He reports no neurologic symptoms or recent skin rash. He occasionally takes ibuprofen for joint pains and has no family history of cardiac disease. An electrocardiogram is obtained (Fig. 40.1) and he is admitted to your hospitalist service. You order a transthoracic echocardiogram, which shows a biventricular dilated cardiomyopathy with a left ventricular ejection fraction of 58% and normal-appearing heart valves.

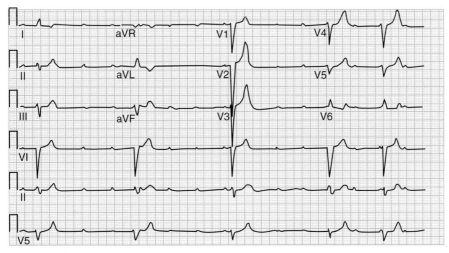

Figure 40.1

Hospital Images: A Clinical Atlas, First Edition. Edited by Paul B. Aronowitz.
© 2012 Wiley-Blackwell. Published 2012 by John Wiley & Sons, Inc.

Question 1

Which of the following historical features fits best with this patient's clinical presentation?

- **A.** Having hiked in rural Connecticut 1 week ago
- **B.** History of a sore throat and a fever 1 week ago
- **C.** An East Coast camping trip 6 weeks ago
- **D.** Having a painless penile ulcer 3 months ago

Question 2

What is the best treatment for this patient's condition?

- **A.** Ceftriaxone
- **B.** Doxycycline
- **C.** Prednisone 60 mg daily
- **D.** Permanent pacemaker placement

Answer 1: C

This previously healthy patient's history of acute onset syncope, new dilated cardiomyopathy, and electrocardiogram showing third-degree atrioventricular (AV) block could be consistent with several infectious etiologies, including Lyme carditis, carditis of acute rheumatic fever, or viral or bacterial myocarditis. Carditis secondary to acute rheumatic fever can include acute heart block but does not appear until 2–3 weeks after the acute streptococcal pharyngitis episode. Despite its recent resurgence in the United States, acute rheumatic fever remains a relatively rare complication, especially in adults.

Primary syphilis commonly causes a single, painless genital ulcer, but late manifestations of untreated syphilis occur at least 1 year after the primary infection and typically occur 15–30 years later. The most frequent cardiac manifestation of tertiary syphilis is syphilitic aortitis, causing aortic root dilation, aortic insufficiency, and heart failure.

This patient's presentation is consistent with Lyme carditis. Lyme disease is caused by the spirochete *Borrelia burgdorferi,* which is transmitted by the *Ixodes scapularis* tick. Infection rates are highest in the northeastern seaboard states (Delaware, Connecticut, New Jersey, and Massachusetts). This patient could have contracted *B. burgdorferi* while hiking in rural Connecticut or on an East Coast camping trip. However, Lyme carditis typically occurs at least 3–6 weeks after the initial infection, making a camping trip the most likely historical feature for this patient. Patients with symptomatic Lyme carditis most frequently complain of palpitations (69% in one case series) but can also report syncope, dyspnea, or chest pain. Disease spectrum ranges from asymptomatic to cardiac tamponade from myoperi-carditis or complete heart block due to conduction system involvement. Although complete heart block occurs in less than 1% of reported Lyme disease cases, it is seen in up to 50% of individuals with Lyme carditis. As in this patient, absence of a history of rash does not exclude Lyme carditis since over 30% of patients with Lyme disease do not recall a prior skin rash.

Answer 2: A

Recommended treatment regimens for Lyme carditis include a 14- to 21-day course of intra-venous doxycycline or ceftriaxone. Patients with asymptomatic first-degree AV block whose PR interval is less than 30 ms can receive doxycycline. Hospitalization and intravenous cef-triaxone are recommended for individuals with significant symptoms, such as syncope, dyspnea, or chest pain, second- or third-degree AV block, or first-degree block with a PR interval of longer than 30 ms. Since heart block can resolve spontaneously and is usually reversible, permanent pacemaker placement is not recommended. Corticosteroids generally do not have a role in the treatment of Lyme carditis.

Lyme carditis presents most frequently as a transient myocarditis with variable degrees of AV block. Electrocardiograms may change significantly over short periods of time. (Figures 40.2 and 40.3 show this patient's electrocardiograms obtained over the first 72 hours after admission.) Conduction disturbances are usually reversible and typically resolve in 3–6 weeks. Although patients with hemodynamic instability may require temporary pacemaker placement, permanent pacemaker placement is generally not indicated. Acute myocarditis occurs in 10–50% of cases, but only about 5% have impaired systolic function. Although valvular involvement frequently occurs in syphilitic or rheumatic heart disease, it is rarely seen in Lyme carditis. Conduction system involvement can be variable and rapidly fluctuating, and patients with PR prolongation equal to or greater than 30 ms can progress rapidly to complete heart block. Even asymptomatic patients with this degree of PR prolongation should be considered for hospitalization for antibiotic treatment and cardiac monitoring.

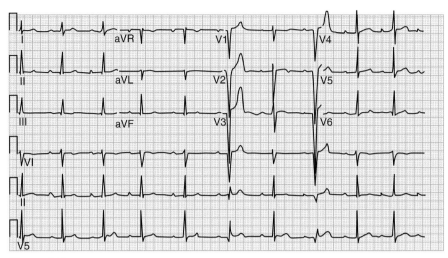

Figure 40.2

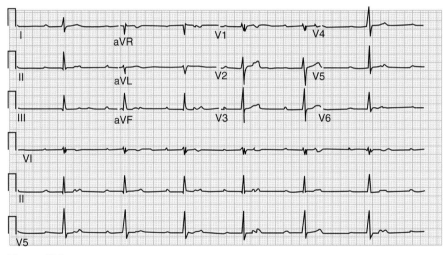

Figure 40.3

FISH AE, PRICE YB, PINTO DS. Lyme carditis. *Infect Dis Clin North Am* 2008;22:275–288.

MCALISTER HF, et al. Lyme carditis: an important cause of reversible heart block. *Ann Intern Med* 1989;110:339–345.

RAMMELKAMP CH, STOLZER BL. The latent period before the onset of acute rheumatic fever. *Yale J Biol Med* 1961;34:386–398.

STEERE AC, et al. Lyme carditis: cardiac abnormalities of Lyme disease. *Ann Intern Med* 1980;93:8–16.

WORMSER GP, et al. The clinical assessment, treatment, and prevention of Lyme disease, human granulocytic anaplasmosis, and babesiosis: clinical practice guidelines by the Infectious Diseases Society of America. *Clin Infect Dis* 2006;43:1089–1134.

Case 41

Image contributed by Alireza Ghotb

A 61-year-old woman is admitted to your service after experiencing hypoxia after a transbronchial biopsy and bronchoalveolar lavage. Her pulmonologist informs you that she has had 5 months of shortness of breath and a 10-lb weight loss but no fevers, chills, sweats, hemoptysis, or history of tuberculosis (TB) or exposure to anyone with tuberculosis. She has never smoked cigarettes. Because she immigrated to the United States from China 20 years ago, he started her on a four-drug antituberculous regimen 2 weeks ago for diffuse nodularity on her chest X-ray. Subsequently, three sputum samples were negative for acid-fast bacilli, with cultures still pending. The bronchoscopy was obtained today because he is still worried about tuberculosis.

You agree to admit the patient to the hospital and continue her four-drug antituberculosis regimen but because her chest X-ray does not reveal a "millet seed" pattern characteristic of miliary tuberculosis, you are suspicious that she may not have tuberculosis. You review the patient's posterior–anterior (PA) and lateral chest X-rays (Fig. 41.1) with a radiologist, who comments on an incidentally noted liver

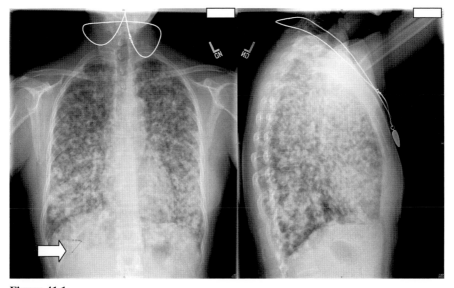

Figure 41.1

Hospital Images: A Clinical Atlas, First Edition. Edited by Paul B. Aronowitz.
© 2012 Wiley-Blackwell. Published 2012 by John Wiley & Sons, Inc.

mass in the right upper quadrant (Fig. 41.1, arrow). You are suspicious that the patient has cancer and obtain a positron-emission tomography–computed tomographic (PET-CT) scan while awaiting results of her bronchoscopy.

Question

If this patient has lung cancer, which of the following is the most likely histologic cell type?

- **A.** Small cell carcinoma
- **B.** Adenocarcinoma
- **C.** Large cell carcinoma
- **D.** Squamous cell carcinoma

Answer: B

Non-small-cell lung cancers (NSCLCs) account for 85–90% of lung cancers. Of NSCLCs, adenocarcinoma is the most common, followed by squamous cell (25–30%), and large cell (10% of all lung cancers). This patient had bronchoalveolar carcinoma, a subtype of adeno-carcinoma, which is less strongly associated with tobacco consumption. As in this case, bronchoalveolar carcinoma tends to have a slightly more indolent course and a tendency to have intrapulmonary metastatic disease. The PET-CT scan you obtained shows metastatic disease in the liver and bone. Magnetic resonance imaging of the brain subsequently reveals innumerable cerebral metastases. This patient has Stage IV bronchoalveolar lung cancer. She still has a reasonable performance status so an oncologist should be consulted for consider-ation of palliative chemotherapy. Several phase III studies have shown that chemotherapy improves overall survival by months compared with best supportive care in patients with NSCLCs. Chemotherapy can also relieve cancer-related symptoms and improve the quality of remaining life, and it is cost-effective compared with supportive care.

ALGUIRE PC (Ed.). *Hematology and Oncology. Medical Knowledge Self-Assessment Program 15.* Philadelphia: American College of Physicians; 2010:80–83.

Case 42

Image contributed by Lauren Friedly

A 46-year-old man with a history of acquired immunodeficiency syndrome (AIDS) is admitted to the hospital for a large, fluctuant left flank mass with an apparently contiguous intra-abdominal fluid collection (Fig. 42.1, arrows). The mass has been present and increasing in size for 3 weeks. The patient has a history of Kaposi's sarcoma, herpes simplex virus infection, and diarrhea with *Mycobacterium avium* complex (MAC) growing in prior stool specimens. One month prior to admission, the patient's CD4 cell count was 17 cc/mm^3 and highly active antiretroviral therapy (HAART) was initiated. His CD4 count is now 218 cc/mm^3. A computerized tomography (CT)–guided fine needle aspiration of the flank mass reveals acid-fast bacilli on acid-fast smear and the material subsequently grows MAC.

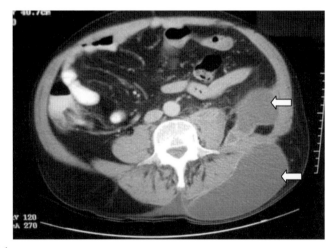

Figure 42.1

Hospital Images: A Clinical Atlas, First Edition. Edited by Paul B. Aronowitz.
© 2012 Wiley-Blackwell. Published 2012 by John Wiley & Sons, Inc.

Question

While reviewing the patient's microbiology results with him, the patient becomes tearful and asks you if he is going to die in the next 6 months. Which of the following would you tell him?

A. He has advanced AIDS and he is unlikely to respond to antimycobacterial therapy.

B. He has a good prognosis but he will need to remain on antimycobacterial therapy for the rest of his life.

C. He has a good prognosis and he will probably be able to stop antimycobacterial therapy in several weeks or months depending upon his response to therapy.

Answer: C

This patient has *Mycobacterium avium* complex reconstitution inflammatory syndrome. Immune reconstitution inflammatory syndrome (IRIS) can occur days, weeks, or months after the initiation and reconstitution of the immune system in HIV-infected patients. The two main types of IRIS are a paradoxical worsening of previously treated opportunistic infections (paradoxical IRIS) or the unmasking of of previously untreated, subclinical infections (unmasked IRIS). This syndrome is thought to occur due to an exaggerated activation of the immune system. IRIS has been associated with a number of diseases, including progressive multifocal leukoencephalopathy, Kaposi's sarcoma, MAC, tuberculosis, non-Hodgkin lymphoma, and cryptococcal meningitis.

To date it is unclear how many patients starting antiretroviral therapy (ART) develop IRIS, but estimates range from 10% to 50%. It appears that the difference in incidence of IRIS in those starting ART is related to the CD4 cell count at baseline prior to initiation of ART; the lower the CD4 count, the higher the incidence of IRIS. It also appears that the incidence is higher in those patients with a history of cytomegalovirus retinitis, cryptococcal meningitis, and tuberculosis.

The overall mortality for patients developing IRIS is approximately 4% for all forms of IRIS, but mortality appears to be more pronounced in those with cryptococcal meningitis IRIS (21%). In general, the prognosis for patients presenting with MAC IRIS is good, with the majority of patients subsequently being able to stop antimycobacterial therapy.

MULLER M, et al. Immune reconstitution inflammatory syndrome in patients starting antiretroviral therapy for HIV infection: a systematic review and meta-analysis. *Lancet Infect Dis* 2010;10: 251–261.

PHILLIPS P, et al. Nontuberculous mycobacterial immune reconstitution syndrome in HIV-infected patients: spectrum of disease and long-term follow-up. *Clin Infect Dis* 2005;41:1483–1497.

Case 43

Image contributed by Estella Geraghty and Bryan Ristow

A 45-year-old woman with a history of rheumatoid arthritis is admitted from the Emergency Department (ED) to your service with fever of 40.2°C and altered mental status. She was begun on a tumor necrosis factor (TNF) inhibitor (infliximab) 4 months ago, and she returned from vacation in sub-Saharan Africa 1 week ago and has had intermittent high fevers since her return. She opted not to take medications for malaria prophylaxis while in Africa. The ED physician has ordered blood cultures and thin and thick (Fig. 43.1) blood smears. Shortly after admission she has a generalized, tonic–clonic seizure.

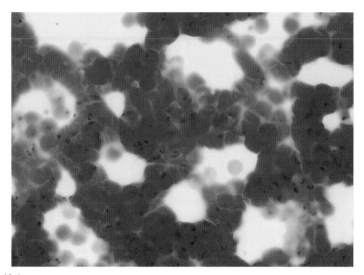

Figure 43.1

Hospital Images: A Clinical Atlas, First Edition. Edited by Paul B. Aronowitz.
© 2012 Wiley-Blackwell. Published 2012 by John Wiley & Sons, Inc.

Question 1

This patient's presentation is most consistent with which of the following:

   A. Cerebral malaria
   B. *Histoplasmosis capsulatum* sepsis
   C. *Streptococcus pyogenes* sepsis
   D. *Listeria monocytogenes* sepsis with meningitis

Question 2

The best subsequent step in this patient's care would be which of the following:

   A. Initiate intravenous therapy with chloroquine and doxycycline.
   B. Begin amphotericin B.
   C. Begin ceftriaxone, ampicillin, and vancomycin.
   D. Begin plasmapheresis.

Answer 1: A

This patient has returned from a malaria endemic region with fevers and was not taking malaria prophylaxis. Although she is at risk of dengue fever, rickettsial diseases, and typhoid fever, malaria should be high on the list and blood smears ordered urgently. An additional complicating factor is that this patient is taking a TNF inhibitor to treat her rheumatoid arthritis. It is clear that patients being treated with TNF inhibitors have an increased risk of *Mycobacterium tuberculosis*, fungal, *Salmonella*, *Listeria*, and *Legionella* infections. The high degree of parasitemia and acuity of illness in this patient are also likely related to treatment with a TNF inhibitor and resultant immune-compromised state. The diagnosis of malaria has been confirmed, as the blood smear reveals characterisitic intraerythrocytic ring forms (trophozoites) associated with *Plasmodium falciparum* infection; *P. falciparum* is the only form of malaria that causes cerebral malaria. The red blood cells that have been parasitized express glycoproteins that are sticky. These glycoproteins ("knobs") stick to capillary walls, causing sludging in the cerebral capillaries. This sludging causes ischemia, capillary leak, and petechial hemorrhages.

Answer 2: A

This patient should be transferred to the Intensive Care Unit for maximum supportive care. The Centers for Disease Control website should be consulted to clarify whether she has travelled in a region with chloroquine-resistant malaria and appropriate antimalarials started. Red blood cell exchange transfusion may also be indicated.

Although consideration should be given to other diseases occurring in returned travelers from abroad as well as to other diseases affecting patients taking TNF inhibitors, this patient's blood smear is consistent with malaria with very high parasitemia. Data from the British Society for Rheumatology Biologics Register found that the risk of serious infection is highest in the first 6 months after TNF-inhibitor therapy is begun and then falls after those 6 months.

FREEDMAN DO, et al. Spectrum of disease and relation to place of exposure among ill returned travelers. *N Engl J Med* 2006;354(2):119–130.

GALLOWAY JB, et al. Anti-TNF therapy is associated with an increased risk of serious infections in patients with rheumatoid arthritis especially in the first 6 months of treatment: updated results from the British Society for Rheumatology Biologics Register with special emphasis on risks in the elderly. *Rheumatology* 2011;50(1):124–131.

GERAGHTY EM, et al. Overwhelming parasitemia with *Plasmodium falciparum* infection in a patient receiving infliximab therapy for rheumatoid arthritis. *Clin Infect Dis* 2007;44:e82–e84.

Case 44

A 41-year-old man is admitted to your service for cellulitis of the left, lower extremity.

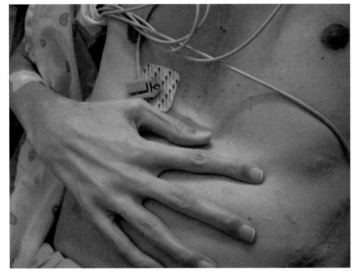

Figure 44.1

Hospital Images: A Clinical Atlas, First Edition. Edited by Paul B. Aronowitz.
© 2012 Wiley-Blackwell. Published 2012 by John Wiley & Sons, Inc.

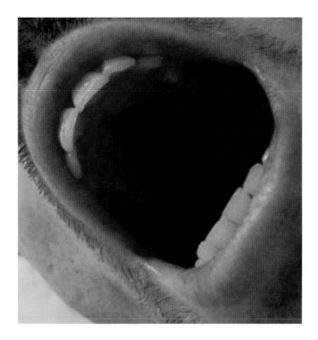

Figure 44.2

Question 1

Which of the following associated clinical features of this patient's underlying condition (Figs. 44.1 and 44.2) puts him at greatest risk of premature death?

  A. Ectopia lentis
  B. Spontaneous pneumothorax
  C. Mitral valve prolapse
  D. Aortic root dilatation

Question 2

Of the following options, which would *not* be recommended to this patient?

  A. Beta-blocker therapy
  B. Regular light weight lifting to preserve muscle tone
  C. Avoidance of strenuous activity
  D. Angiotensin receptor blocking (ARB) agents

Answer 1: D

This patient has Marfan syndrome, an autosomal dominant heritable disorder affecting connective tissue. These images illustrate arachnodactyly and pectus excavatum (Fig. 44.1) and high arched palate with dental crowding, commonly seen in Marfan syndrome. There are numerous other phenotypic features seen in this disorder, including pectus carinatum ("pigeon breast"), scoliosis, joint hypermobility, arm span exceeding height (ratio >1.05), tall stature, and pes planus (flat feet), among others.

The most frequent cause of premature death in Marfan syndrome is ascending aortic dissection. Ectopia lentis (superior lens dislocation), spontaneous pneumothorax, and mitral valve prolapse may also occur in Marfan syndrome.

Answer 2: B

Weight lifting should be avoided in patients with this disorder, as this type of "burst" activity puts additional shear stress on the aortic wall. Strenuous activity should also be avoided for the same reason. There is some credible evidence that both beta-blocking and angiotensin receptor blocking medications slow the progression of aortic root dilatation and should be considered in these patients.

BROOKE BS, et al. Angiotensin II blockade and aortic-root dilation in Marfan's syndrome. *N Engl J Med* 2008;358(26):2787–2795.

PYERITIZ RE. The Marfan syndrome. *Ann Rev Med* 2000;51:481–510.

Case 45

Images contributed by Vanessa London

An otherwise healthy 62-year-old man presents to the Emergency Department (ED) for complaints of headache, fever, chills, and myalgias. His temperature in triage is 39°C and he is completely oriented and appropriate without meningismus. Shortly after presentation to the ED he develops septic shock with a blood pressure of 71/46 mmHg and is noted to have acute kidney injury, leukocytosis, and 38% band forms on his peripheral blood smear. Chest X-ray and urinalysis are normal. Cultures are done and broad-spectrum antibiotics are administered in the ED, and he is admitted to your service in the Intensive Care Unit (ICU) for "early goal-directed therapy." Less than 8 hours after admission you are contacted by a nurse and the intern on the ICU team to evaluate a rash that appeared over 30 minutes (Fig. 45.1).

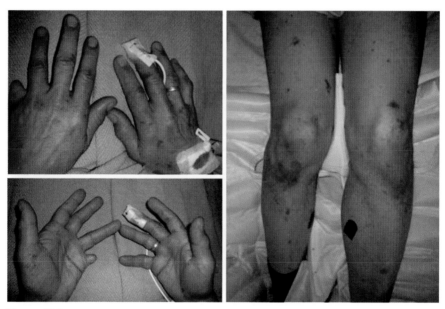

Figure 45.1   New skin lesions arising over 30 minutes, 8 hours after initial presentation to the ED.

Hospital Images: A Clinical Atlas, First Edition. Edited by Paul B. Aronowitz.
© 2012 Wiley-Blackwell. Published 2012 by John Wiley & Sons, Inc.

Question 1

Based upon this patient's rash and clinical presentation, which type of organism do you think is most likely to grow from his blood cultures?

    A. Gram-negative diplococci

    B. Gram-positive cocci in clusters

    C. Gram-positive cocci in pairs and chains

    D. Gram-negative rods

Question 2

Which of the following is a complication of this infectious disease?

    A. Endocarditis

    B. Epidural abscess

    C. Sinusitis

    D. Purulent pericarditis

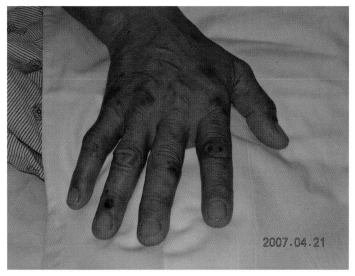

Figure 45.2   Four days after initial presentation.

Answer 1: A

This patient has a purpuric rash (Figs. 45.1 and 45.2) characteristic of meningococcemia. The most common rash of meningococcemia is petechial, but it will often progress to a purpuric rash. *Neisseria meningitidis*, an aerobic, gram-negative diplococcus, can be isolated from the bloodstream in up to three-fourths of affected patients; 50% of patients with meningococcal disease present with meningitis, but somewhere between 5% and 20% will present with meningococcal sepsis without meningitis, as in this patient's case. Meningococcal pneumonia occurs in 5–15% of patients with invasive meningococcal disease. Though staphylococcal (gram-positive cocci in clusters), streptococcal (gram-positive cocci in pairs and chains), and gram-negative organisms can cause disseminated intravascular coagulation and petechiae, this patient's presentation with purpura, sepsis, and no apparent source of infection was more consistent with a rash from meningococcemia.

Answer 2: D

Syndromes associated with meningococcal disease include acute adrenal hemorrhage (Waterhouse–Friderichsen syndrome), purulent pericarditis, pneumonia, epiglottitis, septic arthritis, urethritis, and conjunctivitis. There are also postinfectious complications, which include immune-mediated pericarditis and arthritis. This patient developed postinfectious, immune-mediated arthritis, which responded to treatment with nonsteroidal anti-inflammatory drugs (NSAIDs).

Rosenstein NE, et al. Meningococcal disease. *N Engl J Med* 2001;344(18):1378–1388.

Case 46

Images contributed by Priscilla Yee

Two months prior to admission, an 88-year-old woman presented to her primary care physician (PCP) with a left finger abscess. She had immigrated to the United States from Myanmar more than 20 years ago and did not have any medical problems. She was not a gardener and denied owning an aquarium or pets.

The finger abscess was incised and drained (Fig. 46.1) but failed to heal over the next 2 months despite two courses of oral antibiotics. She then presented to her PCP with complaints of anorexia, low-grade fever, weight loss of 8 pounds, mild cough, dyspnea on exertion, and a neck abscess (Fig. 46.2). She was referred to an ear, nose, and throat surgeon for incision and drainage of the neck abscess. The surgeon noted cervical adenopathy but no epitrochlear adenopathy. Upon incision and drainage, tan-colored purulent material was obtained. The surgeon ordered laboratory studies and a chest radiograph (Fig. 46.3) and has now admitted her to your hospital service and asked you to follow the patient as primary inpatient manager.

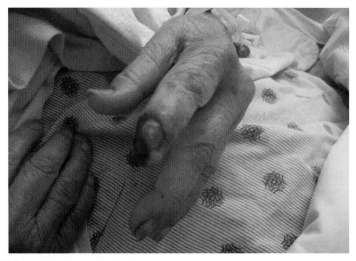

Figure 46.1

Hospital Images: A Clinical Atlas, First Edition. Edited by Paul B. Aronowitz.
© 2012 Wiley-Blackwell. Published 2012 by John Wiley & Sons, Inc.

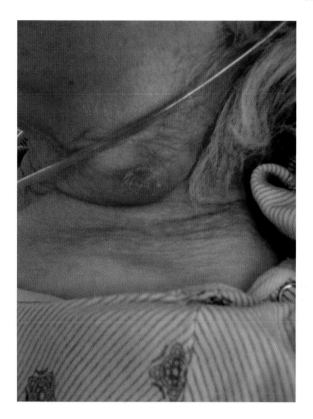

Figure 46.2

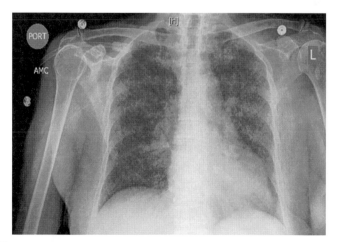

Figure 46.3

Question 1

Which of the following microbiologic tests on the neck abscess drainage material is likely to be the highest yield for making a diagnosis in this patient's case?

- **A.** Gram stain
- **B.** Bacterial culture
- **C.** Acid-fast bacilli (AFB) stain and *Mycobacterium tuberculosis* culture
- **D.** Warthin Starry stain, looking for *Bartonella henselae*
- **E.** Special culture for *Nocardia* species

Subsequently, Gram stain, bacterial culture, acid-fast stain, and culture of both the neck abscess material and tissue from a finger biopsy were all negative. Sputum Gram stain, culture, and AFB smears were also negative.

Question 2

What is the most appropriate subsequent step in this patient's management?

- **A.** Perform an open lung biopsy.
- **B.** Perform an open excision of one or more cervical lymph nodes for pathology.
- **C.** Perform a bronchoscopy with transbronchial biopsy.
- **D.** No further diagnostic workup is indicated; the patient should be started on empiric therapy and observed for improvement.

Answer 1: C

This patient has miliary tuberculosis. Presentations of tuberculosis (TB) are protean. This patient presented with a nonhealing finger ulcer in the absence of other systemic symptoms. There are numerous dermatologic manifestations of TB, including lupus vulgaris, scrofulo-derma, tuberculous gumma, and, as this patient had, cutaneous miliary TB. Her chest X-ray appearance is classic for the "millet seed" pattern originally used in 1790 to describe the small white bumps in the lungs.

Although a thorough history of occupational, hobby, and pet and environmental exposure should be obtained and other diagnostic possibilities considered, this patient's presentation is classic for miliary TB. The term "miliary TB" refers to progressive hematogenous dissemina-tion of tuberculosis. This patient's presentation falls into the category of cryptic miliary TB, as she presented with a prolonged illness with more subtle clinical manifestations. The most likely etiology of this patient's disease is from reactivation TB. Further history revealed that both her son and her mother had TB while she was still living in Myanmar many years previ-ously. Common symptoms of miliary TB include anorexia, fever, cough, and weight loss—all of which this patient had.

Although wound material should be sent for Gram stain and bacterial culture, the higher yield test would be AFB smear and *M. tuberculosis* cultures. The patient does not have a history of exposure to cat scratches or bites, making cat scratch disease (*B. henselae*) unlikely. Cutaneous nocardiosis should be considered in the differential diagnosis, but the chest X-ray finding of a miliary pattern is characteristic of miliary TB and not of nocardiosis.

Answer 2: C

Bronchoscopy with transbronchial biopsy is the best subsequent step for this patient given the miliary pattern on the chest X-ray. Transbronchial biopsy revealed caseating granulomas and acid-fast organisms consistent with *M. tuberculosis.*

Jacob JT, et al. Acute forms of tuberculosis in adults. *Am J Med* 2009;122:12–17.

Fariña MC, et al. Cutaneous tuberculosis: a clinical, histopathologic, and bacteriologic study. *J Am Acad Dermatol* 1995;33(3):433–440.

Case 47

Images contributed by Nhu Chau

The Emergency Department (ED) physician asks you to admit a 53-year-old woman to your service for "some sort of bizarre, bilateral, symmetric skin lesions" (Figs. 47.1–47.3). The ED physician is worried that the patient has a rapidly progressive vasculitis and recommends that you start the patient on antibiotics and consult a rheumatologist. The patient looks well and her vital signs are normal. The patient recently emigrated from Korea and does not speak any English.

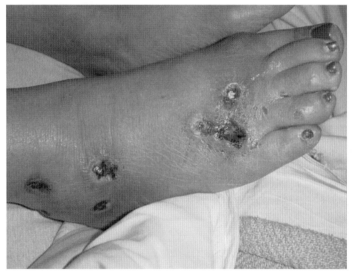

Figure 47.1   Right foot.

Hospital Images: A Clinical Atlas, First Edition. Edited by Paul B. Aronowitz.
© 2012 Wiley-Blackwell. Published 2012 by John Wiley & Sons, Inc.

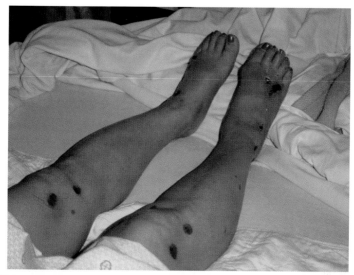

Figure 47.2   Legs.

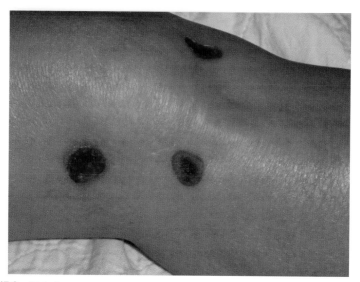

Figure 47.3   Right knee.

Question

In addition to requesting a Korean medical translator in order to obtain a complete medical history, what would be the best subsequent steps in this patient's care?

A. Order erythrocyte sedimentation rate, C-reactive protein, and cANCA studies and start antibiotics.

B. Reassure the patient, counsel her to prevent recurrence of this condition, and discharge her from the ED.

C. Consult Dermatology and Rheumatology, and initiate high-dose steroids while awaiting further recommendations from these consultants.

D. Order hepatitis B and C serologies and serum cryoglobulins.

Answer: B

The lesions seen here are bilateral and symmetric—features that are not consistent with vasculitic skin lesions. Further history obtained with the assistance of a Korean translator revealed that the patient, though untrained in Chinese medicine, had attempted direct moxibustion for intermittent headaches. Moxibustion is a traditional Chinese medical technique that involves burning the herb mugwort (*Artemesia vulgaris*). Moxibustion can be performed indirectly or directly. Indirect moxibustion involves either application of the burning moxa to the end of an acupuncture needle or holding the burning herb close to the skin. With "non-scarring" direct moxibustion, moxa is placed on top of an acupuncture point, lit, and then removed before it burns the skin. With "scarring" moxibustion, the burning moxa is left on the skin until it burns out, leading to burns and scarring, as in this case.

Recognizing cross-cultural treatments different from Western medical therapies is important in avoiding unnecessary testing and treatment. Acupuncture and moxibustion have been used in China and other Asian countries for thousands of years. Studies of moxibustion in supportive cancer care for nausea and vomiting and in inflammatory bowel disease (IBD) have been of limited methodologic quality but generally have not shown moxibustion treatment to be beneficial in IBD or cancer care.

This patient was reassured, educated about the scarring effects of direct moxibustion therapy, advised to keep her lesions clean and dry, and discharged home.

CHAU N. Moxibustion burns. *J Hosp Med* 2006;6(1):367.

LEE MS, et al. Moxibustion for cancer care: a systematic review and meta analysis. *BMC Cancer* 2010;10:130.

MANHEIMER E, et al. Evidence from the Cochrane Collaboration for traditional Chinese medicine therapies. *J Altern Complement Med* 2010;10:130.

Case 48

Written by Susanna Tan
Images contributed by Kjell Jorgenson

A 64-year-old woman with a history of poorly controlled diabetes mellitus, chronic alcohol abuse, and recently diagnosed hemochromatosis is transferred from an outside hospital to your Intensive Care Unit for altered mental status and liver failure. Due to declining mental status from hepatic encephalopathy she is intubated and a nasogastric (NG) tube is placed for gastric decompression; 24 hours later she develops a small area of necrosis at the right naris, and the NG tube is removed. One day later the necrotic area has markedly worsened (Fig. 48.1), requiring urgent

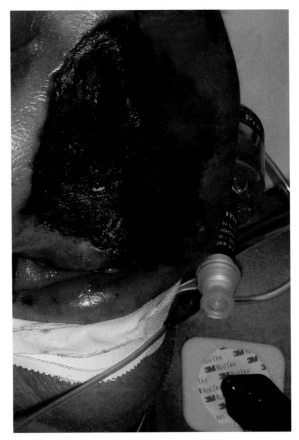

Figure 48.1

Hospital Images: A Clinical Atlas, First Edition. Edited by Paul B. Aronowitz.
© 2012 Wiley-Blackwell. Published 2012 by John Wiley & Sons, Inc.

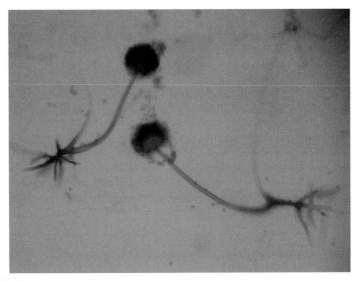

Figure 48.2

surgical debridement. The necrotic material is sent for Gram stain and bacterial and fungal culture. The morning after surgery, the surgeon contacts you for recommendations regarding medical therapy. Bacterial Gram stain and culture are negative. Fungal stains are seen in Figure 48.2.

Question

Which of the following medications would be most appropriate to initiate immediately?

    A. Caspofungin

    B. Amphotericin B

    C. Linezolid

    D. Voriconzole

Answer: B

The patient has rhino-orbital-cerebral mucormycosis. Immunocompromised hosts with poorly controlled diabetes mellitus (especially with ketoacidosis) who are receiving corticosteroids, have undergone transplantation, are neutropenic, or have hemochromatosis are at risk of mucormycosis. This fungus grows extremely well in iron-rich environments—as in this patient with hemochromatosis. Mucorales fungi are commonly found in the air and soil as well as in bread and fruit molds. The broad, irregular, nonseptated, right-angled branching hyphae (Fig. 48.2) are characteristic of fungi in the order of Mucorales. *Rhizopus* species is the most common causative organism, and vascular invasion and necrosis are classically seen in the infective process. Amphotericin B is the treatment of choice. Of the azole antifungal group, posaconazole is most likely to be effective against mucormycosis. Voriconazole and caspofungin are not effective and broadening coverage with linezolid would not be the appropriate next step. The mortality from mucormycosis is high, particularly in the setting of rhinocerebral invovolvement. This patient died within 24 hours of surgery.

SCHECKENBACH K, et al. Emerging therapeutic options in fulminant invasive rhinocerebral mucormycosis. *Auris Nasus Larynx* 2010;37(3):322–328.

SPELLBERG B, et al. Recent advances in the management of mucormycosis: from bench to bedside. *Clin Infect Dis* 2009;48(12):1743–1751.

Case 49

Images contributed by Vinod Raman

A 72-year-old woman presents with complaints of fatigue, nausea, constipation, right chest pain, and left arm pain. The patient denies recent trauma or weight loss. Physical examination reveals left upper arm pain with palpation and right chest pain worsened with palpation of the ribs at the midaxillary line. The Emergency Department (ED) physician orders X-rays of the left arm (Fig. 49.1) and right ribs (Fig. 49.2), which reveal a lytic lesion of the left distal humerus (arrow) and fractures and lytic lesions (arrows) of multiple ribs.

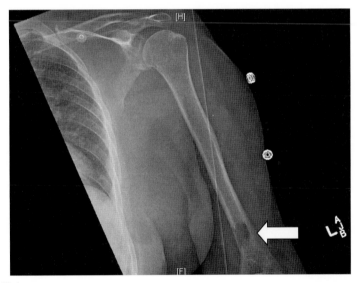

Figure 49.1

Hospital Images: A Clinical Atlas, First Edition. Edited by Paul B. Aronowitz.
© 2012 Wiley-Blackwell. Published 2012 by John Wiley & Sons, Inc.

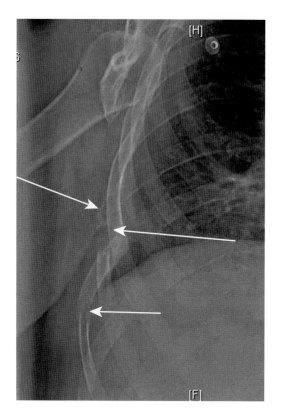

Figure 49.2

Question 1

Of the following, which would be the most likely findings on her laboratory studies?

- **A.** Hyperkalemia and renal failure
- **B.** Hypercalcemia and a normochromic, normocytic anemia
- **C.** Hyponatremia
- **D.** Hyperglycemia and an anion gap acidosis

Question 2

What is the most appropriate subsequent test in this patient's evaluation?

- **A.** Bone marrow biopsy
- **B.** Radionucleotide bone scan
- **C.** Urinalysis
- **D.** Serum and urine protein electrophoresis

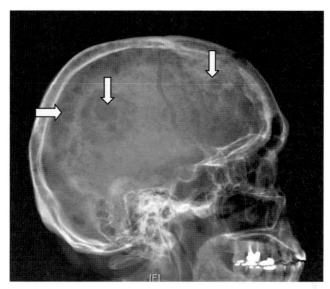

Figure 49.3   Lytic bone lesions (arrows) in this patient's skull.

Answer 1: B

A number of tumors can cause lytic bone lesions, including renal cell cancer, melanoma, non-small-cell lung cancer, thyroid cancer, and non-Hodgkin lymphoma. While this patient's presentation is somewhat nonspecific, the combination of fatigue (from anemia), nausea and constipation (from hypercalcemia), and bone pain with lytic bone lesions puts multiple myeloma high on the list of diagnostic possibilities (Fig. 49.3). Multiple myeloma is one of the most common hematological malignancies in the United States, mainly occurring in older people with a median age of 70 and rarely in people younger than 40 years of age (only 1–2% of all cases). The majority of patients initially present with bone pain or pathologic fractures due to plasma cell infiltration. Other common presenting complaints include fatigue and weakness due to anemia from bone marrow infiltration or renal failure. The anemia is usually normochromic and normocytic. Patients may also present with recurrent infections (especially due to *Streptococcus pneumoniae*) and hypercalcemia.

Answer 2: D

Serum and urine protein electrophoresis along with a complete skeletal bone survey would be the best subsequent steps in this patient's evaluation for multiple myeloma. It is very important to perform the urine protein electrophoresis, as approximately 20% of patients with multiple myeloma do not secrete intact immunoglobulins. In this case the urine electrophoresis will reveal the presence of kappa or lambda light chains. Urinalysis would not detect light chain disease. Bone scan would not be helpful since multiple myeloma causes lytic bone disease, not osteoblastic; bone scans light up in the presence of osteoblastic activity, not osteolytic activity. Bone marrow biopsy should be performed if protein electrophoresis is positive. A minimum of 10% monoclonal plasma cells in the bone marrow and the presence of M protein in the urine or serum are generally required for a diagnosis of multiple myeloma.

This patient had a serum calcium of 15.7 mg/dL, renal failure, and normochromic, normocytic anemia. She was treated with intravenous fluid hydration, loop diuretics, pamidronate, and bisphosphonates, and Hematology was consulted for bone marrow biopsy and further treatment.

Blade J, Rosinol R. Complications of multiple myeloma. *Hematol Oncol Clin North Am* 2007; 21:1231–1246.

Lin P. Plasma cell myeloma. *Hematol Oncol Clin North Am* 2009;23:709–727.

Case 50

Images contributed by Nicole Hickey

While standing on a table changing a light bulb, a healthy 43-year-old man fell, striking his right buttock and lower back; 48 hours later he presents to the Emergency Department (ED) complaining of severe, increasing pain of the low back and right buttock. He is otherwise healthy and has never been hospitalized. His right flank, buttock, and thigh appear slightly mottled (Fig. 50.1). While in the ED he develops a fever of 38.6°C, hypotension with a blood pressure of 80/50 mmHg, and tachycardia with a heart rate of 124 beats per minute. Laboratory studies are remarkable for blood urea nitrogen of 22 mg/dL and serum creatinine of 1.5 mg/dL. His white blood cell count is 10,000 cells per microliter, with 93% polymorphonuclear cells on the differential blood count, and his hematocrit is 40%.

You consult a surgeon, who then makes a small, exploratory incision at the right buttock (Fig. 50.1); a small amount of serosanguinous material drains from the incision.

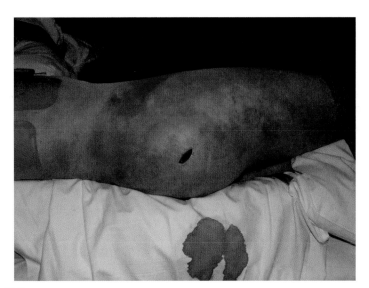

Figure 50.1

Hospital Images: A Clinical Atlas, First Edition. Edited by Paul B. Aronowitz.
© 2012 Wiley-Blackwell. Published 2012 by John Wiley & Sons, Inc.

Question 1

What are the best subsequent steps in this patient's management?

    A. Draw blood cultures, begin intravenous antibiotics, and admit the patient to the Intensive Care Unit (ICU) for "early goal-directed therapy."

    B. Begin aggressive fluid resuscitation, type and cross match in anticipation of blood transfusion, and admit to the ICU until bleeding stabilizes.

    C. Draw blood cultures and begin vancomycin in the ED to cover for gram-positive organisms, and admit to the ICU.

    D. Draw blood cultures, begin broad-spectrum intravenous antibiotics and early goal-directed therapy, and obtain the patient's consent for emergency surgery.

Question 2

Which of the following statements best describes this disease process?

    A. Its histopathologic features reveal necrosis of the superficial fascia with blood vessel thrombosis and suppuration as well as severe subcutaneous fat necrosis.

    B. When it is this severe it involves diffuse hemorrhage beneath the fascia and usually originates from traumatic retroperitoneal hemorrhage.

    C. Its main treatment is supportive and involves fluid resuscitation and red blood cell transfusion as needed but rarely requires surgical intervention.

    D. Though frightening for the patient, it is rarely life threatening and usually does not require hospitalization.

Shortly after admission the third-year medical student on your team asks you what, if any, bacterial pathogens you are most concerned about in this setting.

Question 3

Which of the following best characterizes your response?

    A. You explain that you are not worried about pathogens since blood collections are usually sterile; the issue is intravascular volume depletion due to hemorrhage.

    B. You are concerned about *Streptococcus pyogenes* and, given the proximity to the patient's perineum, mixed anaerobic and gram-negative flora.

    C. You are mainly concerned about *Staphylococcus aureus*.

    D. Given clinical signs of hypotension, tachycardia, and acute renal failure, you are fairly certain that a gram-negative organism is the main culprit.

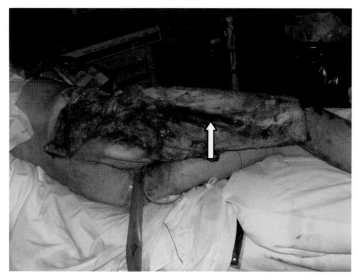

Figure 50.2   Arrow indicates necrotic fascia.

Answer 1: D

Although a hematoma should be considered in the differential diagnosis given his history of trauma, this patient has necrotizing fasciitis. Given that he has no other history of skin disruption such as intravenous drug use or surgery, the most likely etiology is his history of blunt trauma within the previous 7 days. He should have blood cultures drawn, receive broad-spectrum antibiotics with early goal-directed therapy, and be prepared for emergent surgery to debride the involved tissue (Figs. 50.2 and 50.3). The most important treatment of necrotizing fasciitis is surgical. A surgeon should be contacted the moment necrotizing fasciitis is seriously considered. Although a computed tomographic (CT) scan or magnetic resonance image (MRI) of the affected area may be helpful in ruling out other considerations in the differential diagnosis, the diagnosis of necrotizing fasciitis can still be missed with these modalities. Diagnosing necrotizing fasciitis can be difficult and requires a high index of suspicion. Early necrotizing fasciitis is extremely painful, and pain out of proportion to physical findings in a patient, like this one, with signs of systemic toxicity should trigger consideration of necrotizing fasciitis. This patient's fever with signs of sepsis indicates that he has a life-threatening process that is easily located to the buttock, thigh, and low back on visual inspection.

Answer 2: A

The histopathologic features of necrotizing fasciitis reveal necrosis of the superficial fascia with blood vessel thrombosis and suppuration as well as severe subcutaneous fat necrosis. One of the reasons that this disease is easily missed in its early stages is because it involves the fascia while sparing the overlying skin and underlying muscle. Tissue damage is believed to be due to bacterial toxins and local cytokine release.

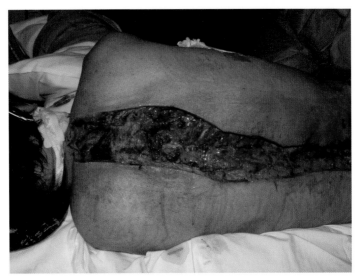

Figure 50.3   Debridement was required from the posterior thigh down to the patient's ankle and as high as the upper back.

Answer 3: B

The goal of empiric antibiotic coverage in a patient as ill as this would be to cover for aerobic gram-positive and gram-negative organisms and anaerobes. *Streptococcus pyogenes* (group A beta-hemolytic streptococci) would be a "bug of interest" given its predilection for causing severe infections in young, otherwise healthy patients. In general, bacterial culture results in necrotizing fasciitis can be divided into two groups. Type 1 is polymicrobial and may involve non–group A streptococci with anaerobes and Enterobacteriaceae. Type 2, also known as hemolytic streptococcal gangrene, is caused by beta-hemolytic streptococci, sometimes in concert with *Staphylococcus aureus*.

This patient was initially treated with early goal-directed therapy, piperacillin/tazobactam with vancomycin, and urgent surgical exploration. Surgery revealed severe necrotizing fasciitis requiring exploration and debridement from the posterior buttock extending to the right ankle and up the back to the upper posterior neck. Blood and wound cultures grew *Streptococcus pyogenes*; after almost two dozen surgeries for debridement and subsequent skin grafting and 3 months in the hospital the patient was discharged home in good condition and eventually returned to work.

GREEN RJ, DAFOE DC, RAFFIN TA. Necrotizing fasciitis. *Chest* 1996;110:219–229.

Case 51

Image contributed by Andrew Cummins

A healthy 81-year-old woman is admitted to your service for syncope, which occurred while she was shopping at a large discount store. An electrocardiogram reveals complete heart block, the patient is admitted to your hospital service, and you consult Cardiology. The cardiologist recommends that a permanent pacemaker be placed and schedules it for the following morning.

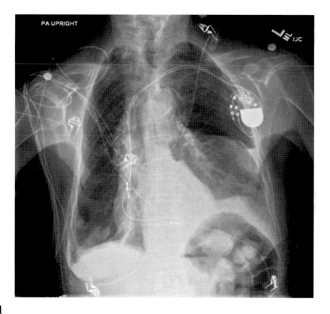

Figure 51.1

Hospital Images: A Clinical Atlas, First Edition. Edited by Paul B. Aronowitz.
© 2012 Wiley-Blackwell. Published 2012 by John Wiley & Sons, Inc.

Question 1

When reviewing the risks of pacemaker placement with this patient, what would you tell her?

A. She has a significantly higher risk of complications than a 50-year-old undergoing the same procedure.

B. She has the same risk of complications as a 50-year-old patient undergoing the same procedure.

C. She has less risk of complications than a 50-year-old undergoing the same procedure.

The following morning a left subclavian approach is used for the pacemaker placement. The procedure is complicated by two inadvertent subclavian arterial penetrations followed by transient hypotension that resolves after the patient is given 1 liter of normal saline via her intravenous line. After completion of her pacemaker placement she is asymptomatic with an oxygen saturation of 98% on room air. A chest radiograph is obtained to assess lead placement (Fig. 51.1).

Question 2

The postprocedure chest radiograph shows which of the following:

A. Mediastinal shift

B. Left pneumothorax

C. Left hemothorax

D. A, B, and C

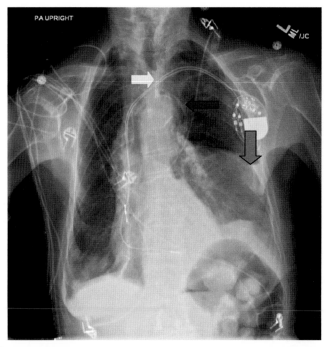

Figure 51.2 Chest radiograph showing mediastinal shift (right-pointing arrow) from left pneumothorax, mediastinal air (left-pointing arrow), and right hemothorax (vertical arrow).

Answer 1: B

There does not appear to be an increased rate of complications of pacemaker or implantable cardiac defibrillator (ICD) placement compared with younger patients in the geriatric or cardiac literature.

Answer 2: D

This patient has suffered two complications of pacemaker placement—a left hemothorax and a partial left pneumothorax. The right-pointing arrow in Figure 51.2 indicates mediastinal shift to the right; the left-pointing arrow, mediastinal air. The vertical arrow points to a pleural fluid collection, later confirmed by a computed tomographic (CT) scan of the thorax (Fig. 51.3, arrow). The patient's hematocrit dropped from 37% at the time of admission to 26% several hours after the procedure. A cardiothoracic surgeon performed an open thoracotomy to remove the organizing thrombus seen in Figure 51.3, and the patient's chest tube subsequently drained 600 cc of blood (Fig. 51.4). The chest tube was removed 1 day later and she was discharged home in good condition 4 days after her admission for syncope.

Complications of pacemakers are generally divided into complications occurring at the time of pacemaker placement, complications related to surgical pockets, and complications related to device function. In the Pacemaker Selection in the Elderly (PASE) study, each of these complications—pneumothorax and hemothorax—occurred in 2% or less of patients undergoing pacemaker placement. The most common complication of pacemaker placement was lead dislodgement, occurring in 2.2% of patients. The second most common complication

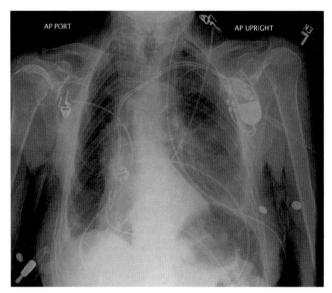

Figure 51.4 Chest X-ray after left thoracotomy and chest tube placement.

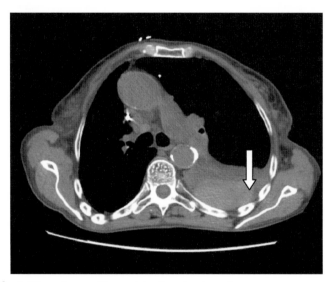

Figure 51.3 Left hemothorax with organizing thrombus (arrow).

was pneumothorax, occurring in 2% of patients. Of note, pneumothorax was more common in elderly patients with body mass indices of less than 20 kg/m^2. Pneumothorax is most often asymptomatic and usually incidentally noted on postprocedure chest radiograph. Hemothorax occurs due to laceration of the subclavian artery during attempts to locate the subclavian vein, as in this patient's case. In addition to lead dislodgement, pneumothorax, and hemothorax, other complications occurring at the time of pacemaker placement include lead perforation of the right ventricle (0.98% of patients in the PASE trial) and vein thrombosis (0.6–3.5% in various studies).

Complications relating to surgical pockets include bleeding, pain at the implantation site, and acute or chronic pocket infections. There are numerous complications related to device function and include extracardiac stimulation, such as diaphragmatic or pectoral muscle stimulation, pacemaker syndrome, and pacemaker-mediated or endless-loop tachycardia.

BAILEY SM, WILKOFF BL. Complications of pacemakers and defibrillators in the elderly. *Am J Geriatr Cardiol* 2006;15(2):102–107.

EISEN LA, et al. Mechanical complications of central venous catheters. *J Intens Care Med* 2006;21:40.

LINK MS, et al. Complications of dual chamber pacemaker implantation in the elderly. Pacemaker Selection in the Elderly (PASE) Investigators. *J Interv Card Electrophysiol* 1998;27:373–378.

Case 52

Image contributed by Eliza McCaw

A 67-year-old man with a history of dual chamber pacemaker placement for complete heart block and a recent pacemaker battery change is directly admitted to your service by his primary care physician. He says he first noticed purulent material draining from an open wound (Fig. 52.1) at his pacemaker site 1 week ago. His temperature is 38.1°C but he is otherwise stable, pleasant, and in no distress.

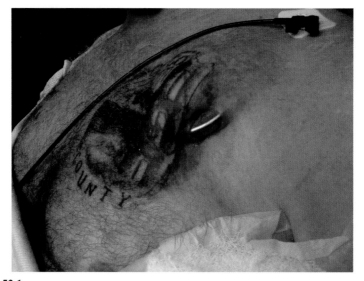

Figure 52.1

Hospital Images: A Clinical Atlas, First Edition. Edited by Paul B. Aronowitz.
© 2012 Wiley-Blackwell. Published 2012 by John Wiley & Sons, Inc.

Question

What are the best subsequent steps in this patient's management?

   A. Initiation of antibiotics to cover for *Staphylococcus* and *Streptococcus* bacteria and Cardiology and Cardiothoracic Surgery consultation for pacemaker and pacemaker lead removal

   B. Initiation of antibiotics to cover for staph and strep

   C. Cardiology and Cardiothoracic Surgery consultation for pacemaker and pacemaker lead removal

   D. Surgical consultation for primary closure of wound

Answer: A

This image illustrates pacemaker erosion due to cardiac device infection. Cardiac device infections are uncommon, with an incidence as low as 1%. Mortality related to these infections is very low (0% in one high-volume medical center in Canada). Risk factors for cardiac device infections include advanced age, a history of device revision or replacement, and multichamber device implantation. Organisms involved in these infections include *Staphylococcus* and *Streptococcus* species. A prolonged course of antibiotics (3–6 weeks) is usually recommended. Therapy also includes removal of lead wires and device as well as separating the explant procedure from the reimplant procedure when possible.

CENGIZ M, et al. Permanent pacemaker and implantable cardioverter defibrillator infections: seven years of diagnostic and therapeutic experience of a single center. *Clin Cardiol* 2010; 33(7):406–411.

McCAW E, et al. Eroded pacemaker in an elderly patient. *Am J Med* 2010;123(3):e5–e6.

NERY PB, et al. Device-related infection among patients with pacemakers and implantable defibrillators: incidence, risk factors, and consequences. *J Cardiovasc Electrophysiol* 2010;21:786–790.

Case 53

Image contributed by Fadi Makdsi and Adam Fall
Written by Joseph P. Henry

You are asked by the Emergency Department (ED) physician to evaluate a 54-year-old man with a history of poorly controlled type II diabetes mellitus who presents with a chief complaint of epigastric abdominal pain. While performing his physical examination he also tells you about a "rash" he has had on his elbows and forearms (Fig. 53.1), abdomen, buttocks, posterior thighs, and knees for approximately 1

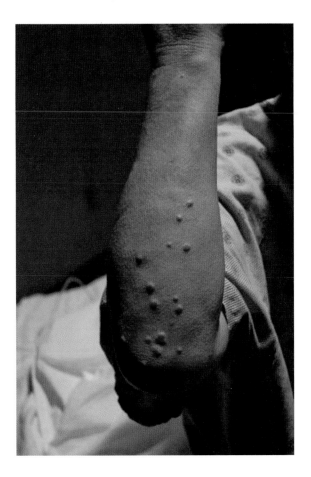

Figure 53.1

Hospital Images: A Clinical Atlas, First Edition. Edited by Paul B. Aronowitz.
© 2012 Wiley-Blackwell. Published 2012 by John Wiley & Sons, Inc.

month. He is moderately tender to palpation in the epigastrium without rebound tenderness or guarding. Laboratory studies are pending and a computed tomographic (CT) scan of the abdomen has been ordered by ED personnel.

Question

Which of the following laboratory and radiologic test results are most consistent with what you would expect to find based upon his chief complaint and rash?

A. Alkaline phosphatase, 451 U/L; lipase, 75 U/L; triglycerides, 175 mg/dL; and abdominal CT scan showing cholecystitis

B. Alkaline phosphatase, 78 U/L; lipase, 852 U/L; triglycerides, 175 mg/dL; and abdominal CT scan showing pancreatitis

C. Alkaline phosphatase, 78 U/L; lipase, 75 U/L; triglycerides, 6200 mg/dL; and a normal abdominal CT scan

D. Alkaline phosphatase, 78 U/L; lipase, 852 U/L; triglycerides, 6200 mg/dL; and abdominal CT scan showing pancreatitis

Answer: D

This patient's history of poorly controlled diabetes mellitus, epigastric pain and tenderness, and the presence of these yellow, waxy skin lesions—eruptive xanthomas—are most consistent with pancreatitis secondary to hypertriglyceridemia. Xanthomas can occur due to primary or secondary hyperlipidemias, and the acuity or chronicity as well as appearance can be clues to the underlying etiology of the xanthomas. Eruptive xanthomas usually precede attacks of pancreatitis related to hypertriglyceridemia by weeks and are an important marker of hypertriglyceridemia requiring medical intervention. With triglyceride-lowering medications and improved control of diabetes, these lesions will usually improve.

Although patients with cholecystitis can present with epigastric pain (rather than right upper quadrant pain), it would be hard to relate this patient's eruptive xanthomas from hypertriglyceridemia to a biliary process such as cholecystitis.

MAKDSI F, FALL A. Acute pancreatitis with eruptive xanthomas. *J Hosp Med* 2010;5(2):115.
PARKER F. Xanthomas and hyperlipidemias. *J Am Acad Dermatol* 1985;13(1):1–30.
TOSKES PP. Hyperlipidemic pancreatitis. *Gastro Clin North Am* 1990;19(4):783–789.

Case 54

Images contributed by Omeed Saghafi, Matthew Crull, and Ian H. Jenkins

A 41-year-old woman is admitted to your service from her primary care physician's office for complaints of fatigue, chronic dysphagia, and a hemoglobin of 4.3 g/dL. Upon admission she reports menorrhagia for several years but review of systems is otherwise unremarkable. Physical examination is remarkable for spooning of the fingernails (Fig. 54.1), angular cheilitis, atrophic glossitis, and conjunctival pallor. Her other laboratory studies show a mean corpuscular volume (MCV) of 48 fL, iron of 6 μg/dL, and a ferritin of less than 1 ng/mL (undetectable).

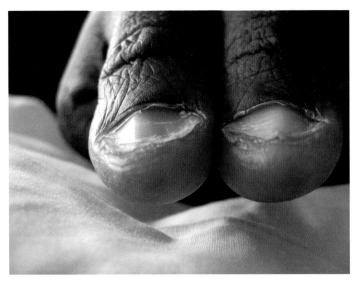

Figure 54.1   Koilonychia.

Hospital Images: A Clinical Atlas, First Edition. Edited by Paul B. Aronowitz.
© 2012 Wiley-Blackwell. Published 2012 by John Wiley & Sons, Inc.

Question 1

Which of the following findings would you most likely expect to find at the time of upper endoscopy?

    A. Esophageal webs

    B. Esophageal stricture

    C. Peptic ulcer disease

    D. Normal esophagus, stomach, and duodenum

Question 2

Treatment of this condition would include which of the following:

    A. Iron replacement and yearly screening for squamous cell carcinoma of the upper gastrointestinal tract

    B. Iron replacement only

    C. Iron replacement and erythropoietin therapy

    D. Iron replacement and administration of a proton pump inhibitor

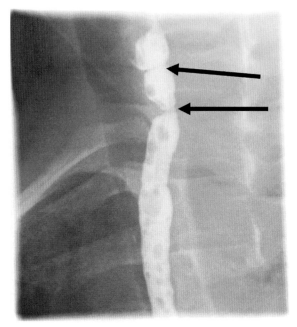

Figure 54.2 Upper esophogram demonstrating esophageal webs.

Answer 1: A

This woman's presentation is classic for Plummer–Vinson (Patterson–Kelly) syndrome. One would expect to find esophageal webs at the time of upper endoscopy. Plummer–Vinson syndrome includes iron-deficiency anemia, esophageal webs (Figs. 54.2 and 54.3), and dysphagia. This disorder was originally described by two laryngologists, Patterson and Kelly, in the United Kingdom in a publication in 1919 but was subsequently also described by two physicians at the Mayo Clinic—Henry Plummer and Porter Vinson. This syndrome occurs in patients with longstanding iron-deficiency anemia but is now very rare due to improved nutritional status and a corresponding decrease in iron-deficiency anemia. Most patients are Caucasian women between the fourth and seventh decade of life. Other physical findings present in these patients include koilonychia ("spoon nails"), angular chelitis, and atrophic glossitis.

The diagnosis is made based upon the presence of long-standing iron-deficiency anemia and the presence of one or more esophageal webs in the setting of dyspahgia. The pathogenesis of this disorder is unknown but appears to be related to iron deficiency. The dysphagia improves in most patients with iron supplementation but in some severe cases, mechanical dilatation may be necessary. The prognosis for patients with this disease is excellent.

Answer 2: A

Iron supplementation is the mainstay of treatment for Plummer–Vinson syndrome. These patients also appear to have an increased risk of squamous cell cancer of the gastrointestinal tract. Though evidence is sparse due to the rarity of this disorder, most literature suggests close follow-up and yearly screening for squamous cell cancer.

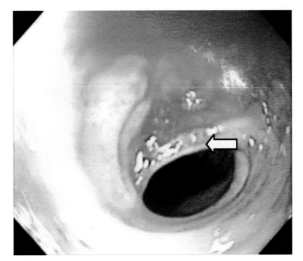

Figure 54.3 Upper endoscopy—esophageal web.

ATMATZIDIS K, et al. Plummer–Vinson syndrome. *Dis Esoph* 2003;16:154–157.

NOVACEK G. Plummer–Vinson syndrome. *Orphanet J Rare Dis* 2006;I:36.

SAGHAFI O, CRULL M, JENKINS IH. Plummer–Vinson (Patterson Kelly) syndrome. *J Hosp Med* 2010;5(5):311–312.

Case 55

Written by Lori Cooper

A 58-year-old male with a history of hypertension presents to the Emergency Department (ED) for worsening swelling and discomfort in his right upper extremity for the past several weeks. He denies any preceding trauma or immobilization of his arm.

Physical examination reveals a middle-aged male in no distress. He is afebrile with stable vital signs. He is noted to have general plethora of his head and neck with a ruddy appearance of his skin (Fig. 55.1). His cardiac examination reveals a regular rate and rhythm without murmurs, and his lungs are clear to auscultation. His abdominal exam is notable for splenomegaly. His right upper extremity is swollen, has a normal radial pulse, and is warm but diffusely ruddy in color (Fig. 55.2). There are also areas of superficial ulceration. Laboratory studies are notable for a white blood cell count of 14,000 cells per microliter, platelet count of 612,000/μL, and hematocrit of 54%.

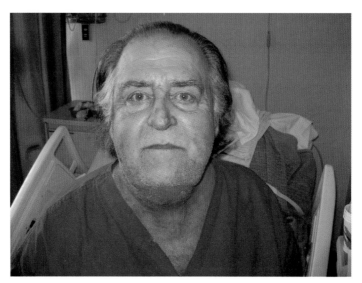

Figure 55.1

Hospital Images: A Clinical Atlas, First Edition. Edited by Paul B. Aronowitz.
© 2012 Wiley-Blackwell. Published 2012 by John Wiley & Sons, Inc.

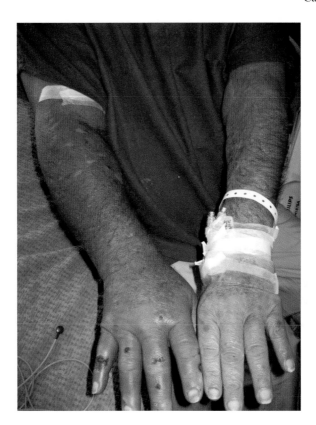

Figure 55.2

Question 1

What would be the best subsequent step in this patient's management?

A. Start intravenous antibiotics for cellulitis.

B. Order a computed tomographic (CT) scan of the chest to look for a pulmonary mass with resultant superior vena cava (SVC) syndrome.

C. Order a right upper extremity ultrasound to rule out a deep vein thrombosis (DVT).

D. Obtain a stat surgical consult for decompressive fasciotomy.

Question 2

In evaluating this patient for his underlying condition, what would be the best next test to order?

A. Obtain blood cultures and cultures of the wound sites.

B. Order factor V Leiden, prothrombin 20210A mutation, anti-phospholipid antibodies, and protein C, protein S, antithrombin III, and homocysteine levels.

C. Order an upper extremity magnetic resonance image (MRI) to assess for deep tissue injury and swelling.

D. Obtain an erythropoietin (EPO) level.

Question 3

In addition to immediate treatment for his acute problem, which of the following would be the best long-term management of this patient's underlying condition?

- **A.** Phlebotomy to a goal hematocrit of <45%
- **B.** Aspirin 325 mg daily
- **C.** Phlebotomy to a goal hematocrit of <45% and aspirin 81 mg daily
- **D.** Lifelong anticoagulation with warfarin

Answer 1: C

This patient has polycythemia vera (PV), which is a chronic myeloproliferative disorder resulting in increased production of red blood cells (RBCs). Generalized facial plethora and ruddy features (Fig. 55.1) are common in patients with PV due to increased RBC mass. Other findings sometimes present on physical examination include splenomegaly, hepatomegaly, and hypertension. Patients may complain of generalized pruritis after taking hot showers due to histamine release from mast cells and basophils. Thrombotic complications include erythromelalgia (a burning sensation accompanied by warmth and discoloration of the hands and feet due to thrombosis of the microvasculature), DVT, pulmonary embolism, stroke, and myocardial infarction. Thrombotic events may occur in up to two-thirds of patients and are considered to result predominately from sludging and hyperviscosity from the elevated RBC mass.

Although cellulitis is a possibility, his leukocytosis is more likely due to PV than an infectious source, and his lack of a fever and cellulitic borders make this diagnosis unlikely. Superior vena cava syndrome can present with facial and upper extremity swelling, but given the presence of unilateral upper extremity swelling this diagnosis is much is less likely. Decompressive fasciotomy is a way to manage compartment syndrome, which this patient does not have.

Answer 2: D

Laboratory studies associated with PV include a hematocrit greater than 52% in men and greater than 47% in women, elevated RBC mass, leukocytosis, and thrombocytosis. Erythrocytosis can occur as a primary disease, as in PV, or secondary to another disorder (e.g., those causing an elevated EPO state such as chronic lung disease, malignancy, or renal cysts). The first step to diagnosis is to exclude a secondary cause of illness; if none is suspected, a serum EPO level should be obtained. If the EPO level is elevated, then the erythrocytosis is likely secondary to another cause; however, if the EPO level is low or normal, then it is consistent with PV. A bone marrow biopsy can be done to further confirm the histologic characteristics and cytogenetics of PV, and a JAK2 mutation can be identified in most patients with PV.

Blood and wound cultures would not be needed in this patient given his lack of fever or obvious infection, as well as the high likelihood of an alternate diagnosis. A hypercoagulability workup is generally not indicated in a patient with a first DVT—particularly given the fact that he has PV. An MRI of the upper extremity would not be helpful.

Answer 3: C

In addition to treating this patient's upper extremity deep vein thrombosis with anticoagulation, he will also need long-term management of PV. The first-line therapy for PV is phlebotomy, with the goal of decreasing blood viscosity and the risk of thrombosis. The goal hematocrit is less than 45% in men and less than 42% in women. Patients with PV should also be on daily low-dose aspirin. Low-dose aspirin (81 mg) is preferred to full-dose aspirin (325 mg) because the higher dose confers a higher risk of bleeding in patients with already dysfunctional platelets from PV. If thrombocytosis and erythrocytosis are refractory to phlebotomy, then administration of chemotherapeutic agents such as hydroxyurea or interferon alpha may be considered. Although this patient will need near-term anticoagulation for his DVT, unless he has repeated thromboses, lifelong anticoagulation is generally not indicated.

LANDOLFI R. Efficacy and safety of low-dose aspirin in polycythemia vera. *N Engl J Med* 2004;350:114–124.

TEFFERI A. Polycythemia vera: a comprehensive review and clinical recommendations. *Mayo Clin Proc* 2003;78:174–194.

Case 56

Image contributed by Sally Daganzo

A medical student on your team pages you and asks you to come to the hematology laboratory to help her interpret a blood smear (Fig. 56.1) performed on one of your patients in the Intensive Care Unit. The patient was brought to the hospital as a "John Doe"—unidentified, found down on a street corner. He is currently intubated, sedated, and unable to give any medical history, and he has never been to your hospital before. He was septic and *Streptococcus pneumoniae* grew from blood cultures within 12 hours of admission. During admission he was noted to have a midline abdominal scar.

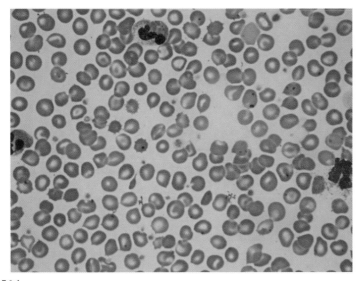

Figure 56.1

Hospital Images: A Clinical Atlas, First Edition. Edited by Paul B. Aronowitz.
© 2012 Wiley-Blackwell. Published 2012 by John Wiley & Sons, Inc.

Question

This smear is most consistent with which of the following:

A. Sepsis
B. Hereditary spherocytosis
C. Thrombotic thrombocytopenic purpura (TTP)
D. Prior splenectomy

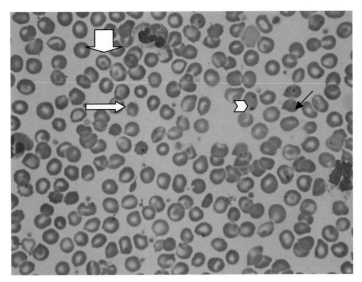

Figure 56.2 Wide downward arrow = target cell; thin right-pointing arrow = burr cell; chevron = Howell Jolly bodies; black arrow = teardrop cell.

Answer: D

This patient presented to your medical center with overwhelming postsplenectomy infection (OPSI). Subsequent history revealed that this patient had had a splenectomy performed 1 year previously, after having ruptured his spleen during a dirt bike riding accident. Patients who have had a splenectomy are at increased risk of overwhelming and sometimes devastating sepsis secondary to *Streptococcus pneumoniae* infection. Whenever possible, these patients should receive vaccination with the pneumococcal vaccine prior to splenectomy and should receive the vaccine every 5 years postsplenectomy. They should also be kept up-to-date on other vaccines against encapsulated organisms.

Findings on this smear include target cells, burr cells, Howell Jolly bodies, and teardrop cells (Fig. 56.2). Howell Jolly bodies are basophilic stained remnant DNA normally cleared by the spleen. There is nothing characteristic of sepsis seen on this smear. A smear in hereditary spherocytosis would show spherocytic red blood cells. A smear reviewed in the setting of TTP would reveal schistocytes and decreased platelets.

OKABAYASHI T. Overwhelming postsplenectomy infection syndrome in adults—a clinically preventable disease. *World J Gastroenterol* 2008;14(2):176–179.

Case 57

Images contributed by Shelley Gordon and Tammy Lai

A 26-year-old construction worker who emigrated from Mexico 11 years ago is admitted from the Emergency Department with several months of cough, fever, chills, anorexia, and weight loss. He reports right leg weakness, which is confirmed on physical examination. A chest radiograph (Fig. 57.1) and magnetic resonance image (MRI) of the spine (Fig. 57.2) are obtained.

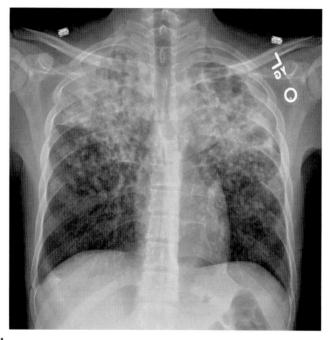

Figure 57.1

Hospital Images: A Clinical Atlas, First Edition. Edited by Paul B. Aronowitz.
© 2012 Wiley-Blackwell. Published 2012 by John Wiley & Sons, Inc.

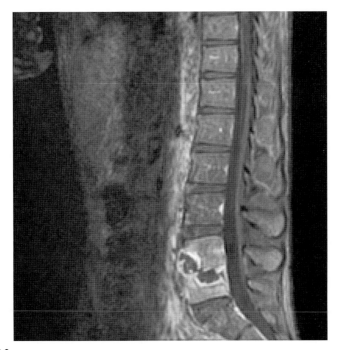

Figure 57.2

Question 1

Which of the following statements is true about this disease?

    A. This is a fairly typical presentation for coccidioidomycosis.

    B. It has a poor prognosis because it is extremely antibiotic resistant.

    C. When involving the spine, it usually begins at the anterior vertebral body at the sub-chondral plate and then spreads to the intervertebral disc and adjacent vertebral body.

    D. Spinal stabilization is virtually always indicated.

    E. This disease usually occurs in elderly patients in sub-Saharan Africa.

Question 2

Which of the following statements is most accurate?

    A. This patient should not be admitted to the hospital as he is highly contagious.

    B. This patient should be placed in respiratory isolation and started on isoniazid, rifampin, ethambutol, and pyrazinamide.

    C. This patient should be placed in respiratory isolation and started on isoniazid until sputum and tissue cultures are obtained.

    D. Little is known about this disease because it was not initially described until 1967 in Lima, Peru.

Answer 1: C

Although fungal infections, such as coccidioidomycosis, would be in the differential diagnosis for this patient, this is a classic presentation of tuberculosis (TB) with disseminated musculoskeletal disease. This patient is an immigrant and presents with typical symptoms of chronic TB, including cough, fever, anorexia, and weight loss. Although musculoskeletal involvement is relatively uncommon (1–3% of TB cases) the spine is the involved site in 50% of cases of musculoskeletal TB. The MRI of the lumbosacral spine reveals involvement of L4, the intervertebral disc space, and L5. Infection of the spine almost always begins at the anterior inferior or anterior superior aspect of the vertebral body; this is thought to be due to better blood supply to this area of the vertebral bodies. It then spreads posteriorly and crosses into the vertebral disc space to involve a second vertebral body. Pott's disease or "Pott's caries" was originally described by Sir Percival Pott in 1782. In TB-endemic countries, this disease tends to occur in older children and young adults. In Western, industrialized countries, Pott's disease tends to occur in immigrants, as in this case, and the elderly. Due to its relative rarity, the diagnosis of Pott's disease is frequently delayed. Spinal stabilization procedures are not always necessary, though this patient ultimately required this treatment due to his neurologic symptoms.

Answer 2: B

Although pulmonary TB does pose a threat to health-care personnel, this patient needs to be admitted to the hospital given his compromised neurologic status. He should be placed in respiratory isolation and begun on a four-drug anti-TB regimen including rifampin, isoniazid, pyrazinamide, and ethambutol ("RIPE"). Isoniazid should not be used alone for active TB, as it may lead to the development of drug-resistant TB. As mentioned previously, Pott's disease was described around 1782 but has been found in the spines of Egyptian mummies, indicating that it has plagued human beings for thousands of years.

LUDWIG B, LAZARUS A. Musculoskeletal tuberculosis. *Dis Mon* 2007;53:39–45.
PERTUISET E, et al. Spinal tuberculosis in adults: a study of 103 cases in a developed country: 1980–1994. *Medicine* 1999;78:309–320.
WARD JW (Ed.). Treatment of tuberculosis, ATS, IDSA, CDC. *MMWR (Morbidity and Mortality Weekly Report)* June 20, 2003;52(RR-11):1–77.

Case 58

Image contributed by Roger Kapoor and Aisha Sethi
Written by Lindsay Chong

A 55-year-old woman with a history of thyroid disease is admitted to your service with a diagnosis of bilateral lower extremity cellulitis. She says that her physician told her she had "bulging eyes" 1 year ago. She says her lower extremity lesions are not painful or pruritic. Physical examination reveals that her lower extremities have a *peau d'orange* appearance with nonpitting edema and hyperhydrosis. Her examination is also notable for exopthalmos, proptosis, and conjunctival erythema.

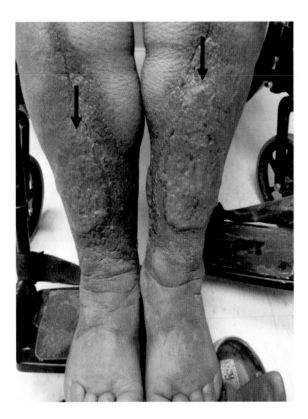

Figure 58.1

Hospital Images: A Clinical Atlas, First Edition. Edited by Paul B. Aronowitz.
© 2012 Wiley-Blackwell. Published 2012 by John Wiley & Sons, Inc.

Question 1

Which of the following is true about these lesions?

    A. They almost always occur after development of Graves opthalmopathy.

    B. They are common skin findings in patients with Hashimoto's thyroid disease.

    C. They are usually painful and puritic.

    D. They are associated with low levels of circulating thyroid-stimulating autoantibodies.

Question 2

What is the recommended treatment for mild forms of this disease?

    A. Intravenous immunoglobulin (IVIG) therapy

    B. Systemic corticosteroids with occlusive local dressing

    C. Topical corticosteroids with an occlusive dressing

    D. Plasmapheresis

Answer 1: A

Thyroid dermopathy (also known as pretibial myxedema) is a rare autoimmune phenomenon occurring in 0.5–4.5% of patients with Graves disease. About 97% of patients with thyroid dermopathy have coexisting ophthalmopathy, which usually precedes development of the skin lesions. The lesions range from flesh colored to slightly pigmented and are most commonly seen in the pretibial area. The lesions may have hyperhydrosis and hyperkeratosis with prominent hair follicles. Overlying skin may resemble the skin of an orange and is described as *peau d'orange* in appearance. The lesions are rarely painful or puritic. The etiology of thyroid dermopathy is not clear, but it is thought to result from the accumulation of hyaluronic acid and chondroitin sulfate in the dermis. Overproduction of glycosaminoglycans may result from fibroblast stimulation from thyroid-stimulating hormone receptors in connective tissue (similar to Graves ophtalmopathy) being activated by high levels of thyroid-receptor hormone stimulating antibodies present in Graves disease.

Answer 2: C

Most pretibial myxedema has only cosmetic importance and does not require therapy. If treatment is necessary, application of topical corticosteroids and occulusive dressing is recommended. A further recommendation is to normalize thyroid function as soon as possible. Systemic administration of steroids, IVIG, and plasmapheresis are used less frequently and usually are reserved for patients who have coexisting severe ophthalmopathy.

Fatourechi V. Pretibial myxedema. *Am J Clin Dermatol* 2005;6(5):295–309.

Kapoor R, Sethi A. Pretibial myxedema. *J Hosp Med* 2010;5(1):59.

Schwartz KM, et al. Dermopathy of Graves' disease (pretibial myxedema): long-term outcome. *J Clin Endocrinol Metab* 2002;87(2):438–446.

Case 59

Image contributed by Anne Fung

An obese 39-year-old woman is admitted from the clinic to the hospital for an initial diagnosis of "severe refractory migraines." The patient is completely oriented and conversant but complaining of headache, double vision, occasional episodes of blurred vision lasting less than a minute at a time, and an intermittent sound "of crickets chirping" in her left ear. She says that when she turns her head to the left the crickets temporarily stop chirping. She denies recent fevers, head trauma, or weight loss. She says that she has gained approximately 5 kg in the past 6 months. She has two healthy children at home. Her right optic disc is shown in Figure 59.1;

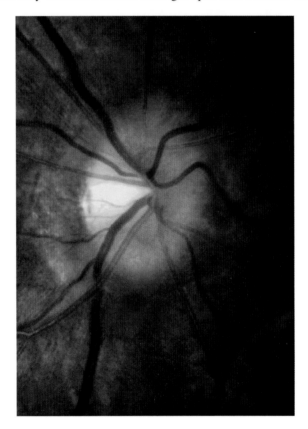

Figure 59.1

Hospital Images: A Clinical Atlas, First Edition. Edited by Paul B. Aronowitz.
© 2012 Wiley-Blackwell. Published 2012 by John Wiley & Sons, Inc.

the remainder of her physical and neurologic examination is normal. A computerized tomographic (CT) scan of the brain (without contrast), ordered by her primary care physician's clinic prior to admission, is normal.

Question 1

What is the best subsequent step in this patient's management?

A. Obtain a magnetic resonance imaging (MRI) study of her brain.

B. Perform a lumbar puncture and check opening pressure.

C. Administer 1 g intravenous methylprednisolone and obtain a Vascular Surgery consultation for bilateral temporal artery biopsies.

D. Begin prophylactic benzodiazepines and obtain a Psychiatry consultation.

A lumbar puncture is performed, which reveals an opening pressure of 35 cm H_2O with clear, colorless cerebrospinal fluid without red or white cells. Protein and glucose levels are within normal range.

Question 2

Of the following, which is the only major morbidity associated with this disorder?

A. Seizures

B. Hearing loss

C. Visual loss

D. Short-term memory loss

Answer 1: B

This patient's history and clinical presentation are consistent with idiopathic intracranial hypertension (IIH), also known as pseudotumor cerebri. Her fundus examination shows papilledema (Frisen grade II with disc margin blurring and circumferential halo). IIH occurs most frequently in young (mean age 30), obese women of child-bearing age. A history of recent weight gain is common. Headache, pulsatile tinnitus, transient visual obscurations lasting as little as 30 seconds at a time, and visual loss are all symptoms of idiopathic intracranial hypertension. Diplopia is caused by sixth cranial nerve paresis. The best subsequent step would be to perform a lumbar puncture and to measure the opening pressure. In obese people, the exact cutoff for the normal upper limit of opening pressure is controversial but is somewhere between 20 and 25 cm H_2O (<20 cm H_2O). Greater than 25 cm H_2O is considered elevated in obese patients.

An MRI of the brain would not add any further information to this patient's evaluation. One gram of methylprednisolone would be the treatment for temporal arteritis, not for IIH. This patient is too young to have temporal arteritis, as she is less than 50 years of age. Her description of double vision and pulsatile tinnitus would also be inconsistent with temporal arteritis.

Answer 2: C

Visual loss is the main morbidity associated with IIH. Seizures, hearing loss, and memory impairment do not occur with this disease. This disorder was first described by Quincke in 1897 shortly after he first introduced the lumbar puncture. It was dubbed "pseudotumor cerebri" in 1904. Foley coined the term "benign intracranial hypertension" in the 1950s, but as more reports of permanent visual loss were recognized, the term "benign" became obsolete. Patients with this disorder should be seen by an ophthalmologist for formal visual field testing and, if abnormal, should be followed regularly as treatment is administered.

One of the most effective treatments for IIH is weight loss—whether by dieting or by weight-reduction surgery. Medication treatments include acetazolamide, which decreases cerebrospinal fluid (CSF) flow, and furosemide, which lowers intracranial pressure. Corticosteroids have been used but side effects (including weight gain) make them a less desirable therapy for long-term treatment. Serial lumbar puncture is controversial, as it only has a transient effect on CSF pressure. Surgical procedures include subtemporal or suboccipital decompression, optic nerve sheath fenestration, and CSF shunting.

This patient's IIH was so severe that, despite trying most nonsurgical treatment modalities, she eventually required a CSF shunting procedure several months after initial presentation.

Ball AK, Clarke CE. Idiopathic intracranial hypertension. *Lancet Neurol* 2006;5:433–442.

Shah VA, et al. Long-term follow-up of idiopathic intracranial hypertension (The Iowa Experience). *Neurology* 2008;70:634–640.

Wall M. Idiopathic intracranial hypertension. *Neurol Clin* 2010;28:593–617.

Case 60

Written by Yile Ding
Image contributed by Brandon Eilertson

You are covering the hospitalist service at night and are called by a patient's nurse who reports that a patient's urine is purple (Fig. 60.1). The patient is a 90-year-old nursing-home resident with dementia who was admitted for hyponatremia and altered mental status. A Foley catheter was inserted on admission and drained normal-colored urine at that time.

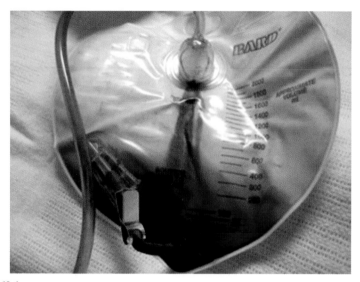

Figure 60.1

Hospital Images: A Clinical Atlas, First Edition. Edited by Paul B. Aronowitz.
© 2012 Wiley-Blackwell. Published 2012 by John Wiley & Sons, Inc.

Question 1

What is the best subsequent step in this patient's management?

   A. Review the patient's medication list and stop the offending agent.
   B. Review the patient's diet and discontinue the offending food item.
   C. Send urine for urinanalysis and culture.
   D. Remove the Foley catheter and change to a different brand of catheter.

Question 2

The nurse is very concerned about the patient's urine color and asks if the purple color is permanent. What would you tell her?

   A. This is a benign phenomenon and will go away with treatment.
   B. This is a benign phenomenon and will go away with treatment, but is likely to recur.
   C. This is a benign phenomenon but her urine will always be purple.
   D. The patient is seriously ill and the etiology of her purple urine is not clear.

Answer 1: C

Answer 2: B

This patient has purple urine bag syndrome (PUBS). First described by Barlow and Dickson in 1978, it is an uncommon but benign phenomenon sometimes observed with alkaline urine in the setting of some urinary tract infections. The urine changes color over a period of hours or days after catheterization, to a range from red or blue to violet or purple.

The etiology of PUBS is still controversial, but most authors believe that the purple color is caused by a mixture of indigo (blue) and indirubin (red) in the urine. The process begins in the gut, where tryptophan is metabolized to indole by gut flora. Indole is then absorbed into the portal circulation and converted into indoxyl sulfate in the liver. Indoxyl sulfate is excreted in urine and broken down to indoxyl by sulfatase/phosphatase-producing bacteria, such as *Providencia rettgeri* and *Klebsiella pneumoniae*.

The prevalence of PUBS ranges from 8.3% to as high as 42.1% in different case series on different populations. Conditions found to be associated with PUBS include female gender, constipation, long-term catheterization, dementia, and diabetic nephropathy. Although associated with the presence of bacteria in the urine, most authors agree that PUBS is a benign phenomenon and does not necessarily need to be treated with antibiotics if the patient is otherwise asymptomatic. One case series demonstrated that PUBS can be prevented by decreasing the duration of catheterization and increasing the frequency of catheter changes.

DEALLER SF, HAWKEY PM, MILLAR MR. Enzymatic degradation of urinary indoxyl sulfate by *Providencia stuartii* and *Klebsiella pneumoniae* causes the purple urine bag syndrome. *J Clin Microbiol* 1988;26(10):2152–2156.

EILERTSON B. Purple urine bag syndrome. *J Hosp Med* 2008;3(5):430.

LIN CH, et al. Purple urine bag syndrome in nursing homes: ten elderly case reports and a literature review. *Clin Interv Aging* 2008;3(4):729–734.

RIBEIRO JP, MARCELINO P, MARUM S, FERNANDES AP, GRILO A. Case report: purple urine bag syndrome. *Crit Care* 2004;8(3):R137.

SU FH, CHUNG SY, CHEN MH, SHENG ML, CHEN CH, CHEN YJ, CHANG WC, WANG LY, SUNG KY. Case analysis of purple urine-bag syndrome at a long-term care service in a community hospital. *Chang Gung Med J* 2005;28(9):636–642.

Case 61

Written by Will Holt

A 42-year-old woman with ulcerative colitis and diabetes mellitus is transferred from the surgical service at another hospital for management of a large abdominal wound and you are consulted. Her colitis has been well controlled with daily oral mesalamine and mesalamine enemas three times weekly. She last required therapy with oral steroids 3 years ago. Three months ago she was begun on insulin because her hemoglobin A1c was 8.3% despite treatment with three oral medications. She had been injecting the insulin into the subcutaneous tissue below her umbilicus. Her abdominal wound started as a purplish papule that quickly progressed to a large ulcerated lesion with heaped-up borders. She has been on intravenous antibiotics since her hospitalization but wound cultures at the outside facility have only grown mixed skin flora. Her wound has continued to worsen despite two attempts at surgical debridement at the outside facility (Fig. 61.1).

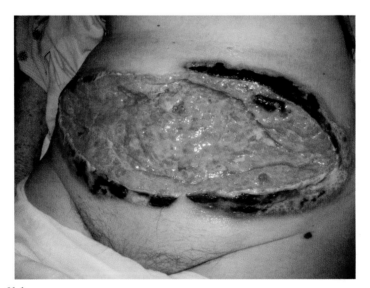

Figure 61.1

Hospital Images: A Clinical Atlas, First Edition. Edited by Paul B. Aronowitz.
© 2012 Wiley-Blackwell. Published 2012 by John Wiley & Sons, Inc.

Question

Which of the following is a true statement regarding this patient's wound?

 A. It is a relatively painless condition.
 B. Skin biopsy shows caseating granulomas with rare nontuberculous mycobacteria.
 C. Corticosteroids should be avoided, as they will worsen this condition.
 D. After complete resolution this wound will recur in up to one-third of patients.

Answer: D

The patient has pyoderma gangrenosum (PG), a dermatologic manifestation of inflammatory bowel disease (IBD) seen in up to 5% of patients with ulcerative colitis (UC) and in up to 3% of patients with Crohn disease (CD). It typically occurs between the ages of 20 and 50 and is slightly more common in women than in men. The disease is associated with a history of trauma to the area of affected skin—pathergy. The lesion begins as a violaceous papule that quickly progresses to a painful ulcer with heaped-up borders.

Pyoderma gangrenosum is a sterile process thought to be due to an aberrant immune response to unidentified factors. It has been hypothesized that the immune system targets its response against antigens that are shared by both bowel and skin. Typically these wounds are sterile but will grow skin flora. Biopsy will show a neutrophilic infiltrate in the ulcer bed and a mixed inflammatory infiltrate at the borders of the wound. Prior to treatment it is important to rule out infectious causes of ulcerating skin lesions, including tubercular, fungal, and bacterial.

Once the diagnosis is strongly suspected, PG should be treated with immunosuppressive therapy. Minor cases may respond to topical steroids but, in cases like this one, systemic steroids are usually necessary. If there is no improvement after 5 days, severe cases may require a second agent such as azathioprine, infliximab, or tacrolimus. Because PG exhibits pathergy, surgical debridement or local injections may make the process worse (as it did in this case.)

Pyoderma is associated with both UC and CD, though it occurs somewhat more frequently in UC. It coincides with the activity of bowel disease in just under 50% of cases. Occasionally, PG will occur before the development of IBD.

Severe cases of PG require many months of therapy to achieve remission. The disease will recur in up to 35% of patients. The ulcerative type of PG shown in Figure 61.1 is more frequently associated with IBD and is more likely to require systemic immunosuppression. In general, risk factors for PG include pan-colitis, black race, and a history of other extraintestinal manifestations of IBD, especially ocular manifestations and erythema nodosum.

BENENTT ML, et al. Pyoderma gangrenosum. A comparison of typical and atypical forms with an emphasis on time to remission. Case review of 86 patients from 2 institutions. *Medicine* 2000;79(1):37–46.

BROOKLYN TN, et al. Infliximab for the treatment of pyoderma gangrenosum: a randomised, double blind, placebo controlled trial. *Gut* 2006;55(4):505–509.

CALLEN JP, et al. Pyoderma gangrenosum: an update. *Rheum Dis Clin North Am* 2007;33:787–802.

FARHI D, et al. Significance of erythema nodosum and pyoderma gangrenosum in inflammatory bowel diseases: a cohort study of 2402 patients. *Medicine* 2008;87(5):281–293.

SU WP, et al. Pyoderma gangrenosum: clinicopathologic correlation and proposed diagnostic criteria. *Int J Dermatol* 2004;43(11):790–800.

Case 62

Image contributed by Sally Daganzo

A 28-year-old man who is visiting California from the Midwest goes camping with his friends. After consuming several cans of cold beer, the man rearranges some boulders around their campsite and encounters a rattlesnake. He is concerned about the snake being close to their campsite and attempts to pick up the snake in order to move it to another location. As he tries to pick up the snake, it coils, rattles, and then bites him on the right second digit.

The man comes to the Emergency Department (ED) at your hospital in Northern California and you are contacted for medical consultation by the ED staff. The man is otherwise healthy but complains of severe pain at the site of the bite, nausea, perioral paresthesias, weakness, and a "strange minty taste" in his mouth. His vital signs are stable except for a pulse rate of 104 beats per minute. Routine laboratory studies, prothrombin time, partial thromboplastin time, fibrin split products, and fibrinogen are all within their normal ranges. His finger continues to swell and become more painful during his first hour in the ED (Fig. 62.1).

The man is anxious and says, "Doctor, please call my family in Wisconsin because I think I'm going to die—I've been bitten by a poisonous snake! What do you think my chances are?"

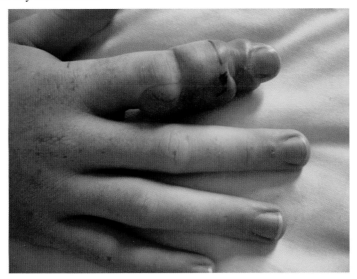

Figure 62.1

Hospital Images: A Clinical Atlas, First Edition. Edited by Paul B. Aronowitz.
© 2012 Wiley-Blackwell. Published 2012 by John Wiley & Sons, Inc.

Question 1

How would you respond to this patient?

- **A.** Mortality from this type of bite is approximately 50% over the next 24 hours.
- **B.** Of an estimated 7000 venomous snake bites each year in the United States, only 5 or 6 result in death.
- **C.** Since it appears he has received an envenomated bite, his expected mortality is approximately 5–25%.
- **D.** His bite appears to have been "dry" (no venom was injected) and with good wound care his chance of dying is close to zero.

Question 2

Of the following, which is *not* typically associated with bites by venomous snakes in the United States:

- **A.** Male gender
- **B.** Employment in landscaping, construction, or ranching jobs
- **C.** Age between 17 and 27 years
- **D.** Alcohol consumption
- **E.** Deliberate attempt to handle, harm, or kill the snake

Question 3

What is the best subsequent step in the treatment of this patient?

- **A.** Administer antivenom in the ED, admit to the hospital, and follow coagulopathy laboratory results closely.
- **B.** Report this case to the County Health Department in your county, and advise the ED physician to observe the patient for 6 hours in the ED and then discharge him home if repeat laboratory studies and vital signs are normal.
- **C.** Admit to the Intensive Care Unit and observe for clinical worsening and consideration of administration of antivenom.
- **D.** Initiate intravenous antibiotics to prevent wound infection and admit to the hospital for 24-hour observation and periodic laboratory studies, including prothrombin time, partial thromboplastin time, fibrin degradation products, and fibrinogen.

Answer 1: B

Of an estimated 7000–8000 venomous snake bites each year in the United States, only 5 or 6 result in death. Eastern and Western diamondback rattlesnakes are responsible for most fatalities. After the introduction of antivenom in the United States in 1954, mortality declined from an estimated 5–25% in the 19th century to less than 0.5% today; 25% of pit viper bites (rattlesnakes, copperheads, coral snakes, etc.) are "dry" bites—no venom is actually injected by the snake. It is very important to clarify whether a victim has been envenomated because panic symptoms (nausea, dizziness, perioral paresthesia, tachycardia) can mimic signs of envenomation. Many venomous snake bite victims believe they are going to die.

This patient probably has been envenomated since he has a classic hemorrhagic bullous lesion at the bite site. He is complaining of a "strange minty taste" in his mouth, which is a symptom associated with envenomation. Other descriptions of this peculiar dysgeusia are as metallic or rubbery. Severe systemic effects can also include tachypnea, altered mental status, respiratory distress, and severe tachycardia. Bites can result in a consumptive coagulopathy and hemolysis that may not be present upon initial presentation.

Answer 2: B

Few venomous snake bites are now associated with agricultural or other outdoor jobs. The vast majority of snake bites (98%) occur on the extremities—usually upper—and result from deliberate attempts to handle, harm, or kill the snake. Most victims are male between the ages of 17 and 27, and alcohol intoxication is a factor in many bites.

Given the elimination of many rattlesnakes in the eastern United States, the majority of bites in the United States occur in the southwestern United States. A growing number of snake bites also result from deliberate exposure to captive native and non-native snakes, such as cobras.

Answer 3: A

Since it appears this patient has systemic signs of envenomation, it would be reasonable to administer antivenom. Unfortunately, indications for the use of antivenom have not been well defined in the United States so much is left to the discretion of the treating physician. If available, a poison control center can be consulted for advice. In the case of rattlesnake bites, progressive effects of the envenomation (worsening local injury, coagulopathy, systemic effects) should prompt administration of antivenom. Antivenom binds venom components and can reverse the venom's effects. Administration should not be automatic to any victim of a pit viper bite since antivenom, products of animal serum, can cause adverse reactions ranging from rash to death. Anaphylactic reactions may occur, and the incidence of serum sickness ranges from 16% to 86% depending upon the type of antivenom administered to the victim.

Snake bites do not need to be reported to county health departments and snake bites rarely lead to wound infections if properly cleansed and cared for. Prophylactic antibiotics are generally not recommended in this setting.

GOLD BS, DART RC, BARISH RA. Bites of venomous snakes. *N Engl J Med* 2002;347(5):347–356.
LEVINE M, RUHA A. Rattlesnake envenomation. *N Engl J Med* 2010;362(23):2212.

Case 63

A 72-year-old woman is admitted to your service for melena and anemia due to a bleeding duodenal ulcer. Her physical examination is remarkable for firm, nontender nodules over the extensor surfaces of her hands and forearms.

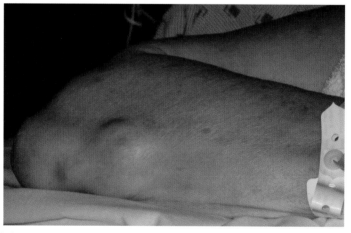

Figure 63.1

Hospital Images: A Clinical Atlas, First Edition. Edited by Paul B. Aronowitz.
© 2012 Wiley-Blackwell. Published 2012 by John Wiley & Sons, Inc.

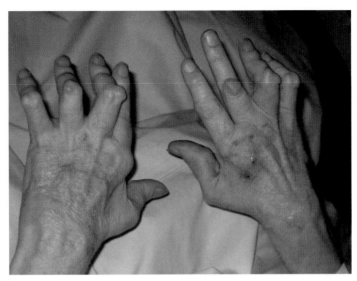

Figure 63.2

Question

Of the following, which statement is *not* true regarding the nodules (Figs. 63.1 and 63.2):

A. These skin lesions are the most common extra-articular feature of her underlying rheumatological disorder.

B. These lesions are one of seven classification criteria for this patient's rheumatological disorder.

C. As this disease progresses, these lesions frequently become infected due to ulceration.

D. These lesions can occur in the vocal cords, nose, lungs, peritoneum, and pleura.

Answer: C

This patient has rheumatoid nodules, the most common extra-articular manifestation of rheumatoid arthritis (RA). These nodules, composed of discrete granulomas in different stages of development separated by scar tissue, occur in approximately 25% of patients with RA.

They are mostly benign and usually do not require surgical intervention or steroid injection. In fact, intervention to excise or inject these lesions may lead to further complications. They usually occur in areas of the body prone to repetitive irritation, such as the extensor surfaces of the forearm, fingers, sacrum, back, and heel. They can also occur in the bridge of the nose at the point of contact with eyeglasses as well as internally in the lungs, pleura, vocal cords, peritoneum, dura, heart, and pericardium.

The seven classification criteria for RA are as follows:

Morning stiffness lasting > 1 hour

Arthritis of three or more joint areas

Symmetric arthritis

Arthritis of hand joints (proximal interphalangeal or metacarpophalangeal)

Subcutaneous rheumatoid nodules

Positive rheumatoid factor

Radiographic changes

In the presence of four or more of these criteria, the sensitivity and specificity for the diagnosis of RA is 90%. Of note, 90% or more of patients with rheumatoid nodules are rheumatoid factor positive.

ARNETT FC, et al. The American Rheumatism Association 1987 revised criteria for the classification of rheumatoid arthritis. *Arthritis Rheum* 1988;31:315–324.

SAYAH A, ENGLISH JC. Rheumatoid arthritis: a review of the cutaneous manifestations. *J Am Acad Dermatol* 2005;53:191–209.

YAMAMOTO T. Cutaneous manifestations associated with rheumatoid arthritis. *Rheumatol Int* 2009;29:979–988.

Case **64**

Images contributed by Tarek Darwish and David Wooldridge

A 32-year-old man presents with complaints of pain and swelling in the right knee and left hand, along with a skin rash on both feet. Physical examination reveals a right knee effusion and dactylitis manifested by both swelling of the digits of the left hand and finger-tip ulcerations (Fig. 64.1), as well as hyperkeratotic plaques with erythematous bases on the soles of both feet (Fig. 64.2). Scaly erythematous lesions over the penis and the scrotum are also noted on genitalia examination (Fig. 64.3).

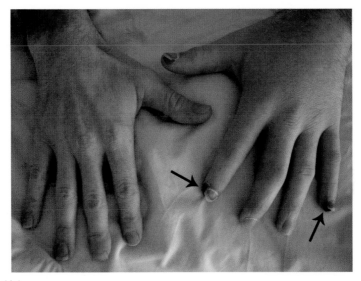

Figure 64.1

Hospital Images: A Clinical Atlas, First Edition. Edited by Paul B. Aronowitz.
© 2012 Wiley-Blackwell. Published 2012 by John Wiley & Sons, Inc.

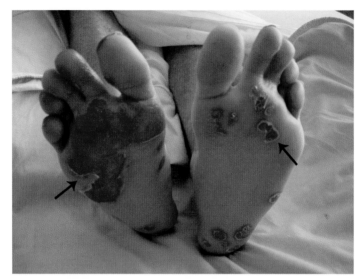

Figure 64.2

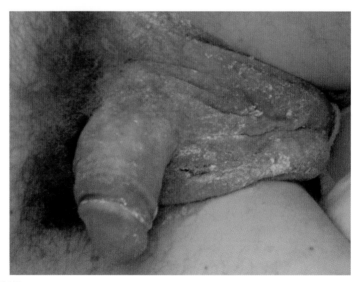

Figure 64.3

Question 1

Of the following, which is associated with this condition?

    A. *Hemophilus influenza* pneumonia 1 month ago

    B. Meningococcal meningitis as a child

    C. *Chlamydia trachomatis* urethritis 2 weeks ago

    D. Rheumatoid arthritis

Question 2

When reviewing the prognosis of this disease with the patient, what would you tell him?

   A. Prognosis is poor, with nearly 100% chance that he will suffer debilitating arthritis for the rest of his life.

   B. Fifty percent of patients will have complete resolution of symptoms by 6 months and the rest will develop chronic remitting disease.

   C. Besides nonsteroidal anti-inflammatory drugs (NSAIDs) and corticosteroids there are no other treatment alternatives for this disease.

   D. You are surprised that he has developed this disorder since he is male.

Answer 1: C

This patient has arthritis, circinate balinitis, and keratoderma blennorrhagicum—all consistent with a diagnosis of reactive arthritis. The classic triad of reactive arthritis is conjunctivitis, urethritis, and arthritis ("can't see, can't pee, can't climb a tree"), but it is increasingly recognized that these three clinical features frequently do not occur together. The symptoms of reactive arthritis usually occur 1–4 weeks after initial infection with a gram-negative bacteria with a lipopolysaccharide component in its cell walls. Pathogens that have been definitely linked to reactive arthritis include *Chlamydia trachomatis*, *Salmonella*, *Shigella*, *Campylobacter*, and *Yersinia*, but there are many other agents that are probable or possible causative agents. The probable causes include *Chlamydia pneumoniae* and *Ureaplasma urealyticum*, while possible causes include infectious agents as diverse as *Clostridium difficile* and *Borrelia burgdorferi*, the causative bacterium of Lyme disease.

In 1916, Hans Reiter, a German physician, described the triad of arthritis, urethritis, and conjunctivitis in a German soldier after an episode of bloody diarrhea. Since he mistakenly thought this syndrome was caused by a spirochete, he named it spirochetosis arthritica. The syndrome was named after Reiter in 1942 by two Harvard researchers, but subsequently the name was changed to reactive or postinfectious arthritis because Reiter had authorized experiments on German concentration camp prisoners and was therefore not felt to be deserving of having a syndrome named after him.

Answer 2: B

Approximately 50% of patients developing reactive arthritis will have spontaneous resolution of their symptoms within 6 months, while the other 50% develop chronic reactive arthritis. Treatment for reactive arthritis includes NSAIDs, corticosteroids, and disease-modifying antirheumatic drugs. NSAIDs help with the arthritic aspects of the disease but not with the mucocutaneous or ocular pathology. Tumor necrosis factor (TNF) inhibitors have been tried in some patients for whom traditional therapies fail, and this patient ultimately required therapy with these agents due to severe, chronic remitting symptoms.

CARTER JD. Reactive arthritis: defined etiologies, emerging pathophysiology, and unresolved treatment. *Infect Dis Clin North Am* 2006;20:827–847.

DARWISH T, WOOLDRIDGE D. Thirty-two-year-old male with arthritis and a scaly skin rash. *J Hosp Med* 2009;4(6):390.

WU IB, SCHWARTZ RA. Rieter's syndrome: the classic triad and more. *J Am Acad Dermatol* 2008; 59:113–121.

Case 65

Written by Susanna Tan

A 59-year-old real estate developer who owns a remote, rustic cabin in the Sierra Nevada Mountains in California and has recently traveled to Mexico is admitted from the Emergency Department to your service with intermittent episodes of fever. He says he and his wife became ill with fever 1 month ago and she recovered completely after 1 week. He defervesced after 1 week and his fever recurred about 1 week later. After several days of high fevers and rigors, he again defervesced. He was without symptoms for several days and now he is on his third stretch of fevers, with a fever this evening of 40.2°C. Other than myalgias and mild headache only when febrile, he has no other specific complaints. The patient adamantly denied having been bitten by insects while in Mexico or while visiting his cabin in the mountains approximately 1 month previously. Concerned that the patient could have contracted malaria while in Mexico, the medical resident on your team has ordered thick and thin (Fig. 65.1) blood smears.

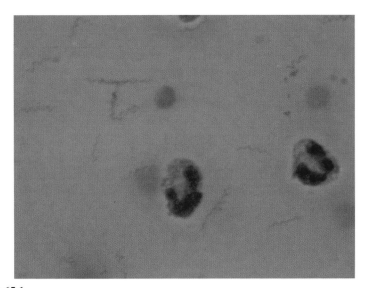

Figure 65.1

Hospital Images: A Clinical Atlas, First Edition. Edited by Paul B. Aronowitz.
© 2012 Wiley-Blackwell. Published 2012 by John Wiley & Sons, Inc.

Question 1

Which vector did the patient most likely come into contact with?

    A. Anopheles mosquito

    B. Sand fly

    C. Tsetse fly

    D. Soft tick

Question 2

After receiving intravenous doxycycline, the patient develops fever, tachycardia, hypotension, flushing, and rigors. What is the best subsequent step in this patient's management?

    A. Change antibiotics to amphotericin B.

    B. Add a cephalosporin antibiotic since he is likely to be co-infected with another infectious agent.

    C. Continue doxycycline and supportive care.

    D. Stop doxycycline and switch to a cephalosporin antibiotic—he is allergic to doxycycline.

Answer 1: D

This patient has tick-borne relapsing fever. The smear shows spirochetes, characteristic of the genus *Borrelia*, which is transmitted to humans through the bite of soft ticks from the genus *Ornithodoros*. The *Anopheles* mosquito transmits *Plasmodium falciparum*, which causes malaria in humans. The tsetse fly is the vector for African trypanosomiasis ("sleeping sickness"). Leishmaniasis is transmitted by the bite of the sand fly.

This patient became infected with *Borrelia* while visiting his cabin in the mountains. Soft ticks live on ground squirrels, which are abundant underneath and around his cabin. Since soft ticks feed at night and only need to feed on a victim for 15 to 30 minutes to transmit the disease, it is not surprising that the patient did not recall being bitten.

Answer 2: C

This patient is having a Jarisch–Herxheimer reaction, which occurs in approximately 50% of patients treated for relapsing fever. It occurs within the first few hours after initiation of treatment and usually resolves within 24 hours. The Jarisch–Herxheimer reaction is often associated with fever, malaise, myalgias, headache, chills, tachycardia, increased respiratory rate, and hemodynamic instability. The reaction is thought to be due to liberation of antigens from spirochetes leading to activation of the complement system. Treatment is supportive and includes intravenous fluids and antipyretics.

DWORKIN MS, et al. Tick-borne relapsing fever. *Infect Dis Clin North Am* 2008;22(3):449–468.

GRIFFIN GE. Cytokines involved in human septic shock—the model of the Jarisch–Herxheimer reaction. *J Antimicrob Chemother* 1998;41(Suppl A):25–29.

ROSCOE C, EPPERLY T. Tick-borne relapsing fever. *Am Fam Phys* 2005;72(10):2039–2044.

Case **66**

Written by Vanessa London
Images contributed by Vanessa London and David Peng

A 45-year-old woman with a history of endocarditis and intravenous drug use is admitted from the Emergency Department (ED) with shortness of breath and complaints of a rash (Fig. 66.1) for 3 days. Evaluation in the ED reveals a fever of 40.2°C and hypotension as well as leukocytosis and acute kidney injury on laboratory testing.

Her heart rate is 126 beats per minute, and you believe that you hear a holosystolic murmur at the cardiac apex that radiates to the axilla. Dermatology is consulted and a punch biopsy of one of her skin lesions is performed. Initial pathology reveals

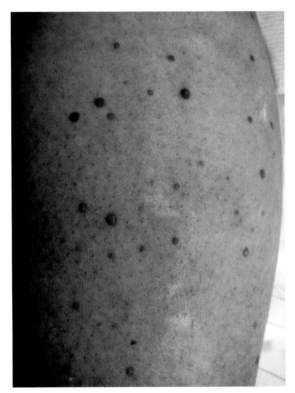

Figure 66.1 Posterior lower leg.

Hospital Images: A Clinical Atlas, First Edition. Edited by Paul B. Aronowitz.
© 2012 Wiley-Blackwell. Published 2012 by John Wiley & Sons, Inc.

clusters of gram-positive cocci and culture grows *Staphylococcus aureus* within 12 hours.

Question

What is the most likely diagnosis?

A. Acute bacterial endocarditis
B. Subacute bacterial endocarditis
C. Acute rheumatic fever
D. Necrotizing fasciitis

Answer: A

With a history of endocarditis and intravenous drug use, stigmata of septic emboli on the skin, multiorgan involvement, and rapid decompensation, this patient most likely has acute bacterial endocarditis. Previous endocarditis is one of the most important risk factors for endocarditis in this patient, but her use of injection drugs alone places her at approximately 30 times the risk of endocarditis as the general population. Her heart murmur at the time of admission was indicative of involvement of the mitral valve. The most common site of endocarditis in intravenous drug users is the tricuspid valve, but involvement of the mitral valve occurs in about one-fourth of cases.

Staphylococcus aureus is a typical organism in the setting of acute infectious endocarditis, whereas Streptococcus species would be more typical organisms in subacute infectious endocarditis. This patient subsequently died from overwhelming sepsis, with Staphylococcus aureus growing from multiple blood cultures and pleural and cerebrospinal fluids.

MATTHEW J, ADDAI T, ANAND A, et al. Clinical features, site of involvement, bacteriologic findings, and outcome of infective endocarditis in intravenous drug users. *Arch Intern Med* 1995;155(15): 1641–1648.

SAYDAIN G, SINGH J, BHAVINKUMAR D, et al. Outcome of patients with injection drug use—associated endocarditis admitted to an intensive care unit. *J Crit Care* 2010;25:248–253.

Case 67

Written by Joseph P. Henry

A 62-year-old man who has not seen a doctor in 10 years is admitted to the hospital with nausea, vomiting, and severe epigastric pain that began 10 hours prior to admission. The pain is worse with eating and radiates to the back. He has a family history of diabetes, drinks two cans of beer daily, and does not smoke tobacco. Physical examination is notable for moderate epigastric tenderness with palpation. You are contacted by nursing staff to evaluate the patient shortly after admission because the phlebotomist is concerned "there is pus in the patient's blood" (Fig. 67.1).

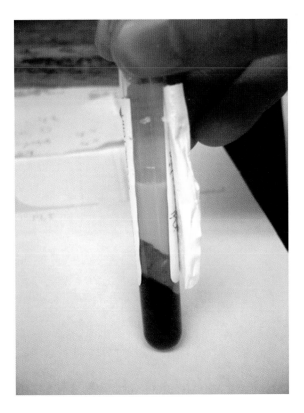

Figure 67.1

Hospital Images: A Clinical Atlas, First Edition. Edited by Paul B. Aronowitz.
© 2012 Wiley-Blackwell. Published 2012 by John Wiley & Sons, Inc.

Question

What is the most likely diagnosis?

- **A.** Gram-negative sepsis
- **B.** Acute pancreatitis
- **C.** Cholecystitis
- **D.** Diabetic ketoacidosis

Answer: A

This patient has acute pancreatitis secondary to hypertriglyceridemia. His serum triglyceride level was 5170 mg/dL and lipase was 356 U/L. Hypertriglyceridemia is the third most common cause of acute pancreatitis after alcohol and gallstones. It is more likely to occur when triglycerides exceed 1000 mg/dL but can occasionally be seen with triglycerides between 500 and 1000 mg/dL. This image illustrates the separation of the chylomicrons that form in the serum making it latescent (milky coloration).

There are various causes of hypertriglyceridemia, with the most common being poorly controlled type II diabetes followed by genetic defects in the production or metabolism of triglycerides. Several cases have also been reported in the setting of binge drinking and pregnancy. This patient was found to have type II diabetes mellitus.

Regarding treatment of hypertriglyceridemic pancreatitis, in multiple small trials, apheresis has decreased symptoms and shortened hospital stay but has not decreased mortality in patients with severe pancreatitis. This patient should also receive aggressive fluid resuscitation, he should not be given anything by mouth, and, if his glucose is greater than 500 mg/dL, an intravenous insulin drip should be strongly considered. Insulin decreases serum triglyceride levels by enhancing lipoprotein lipase activity, which breaks down chylomicrons. Heparin has also been used in this setting, as it stimulates the release of endothelial lipoprotein lipase into the circulation. Various authors have reported the use of heparin along with insulin to treat hypertriglyceridemia-induced pancreatitis. Oral triglyceride-lowering agents, such as gemfibrizol, should also be intitated as soon as the patient is able to tolerate oral therapy.

KYRIAKIDIS AV, et al. Management of acute severe hyperlipidemic pancreatitis. *Digestion* 2006; 73(4):259-264.

Case 68

A 67-year-old man is admitted to your service for fatigue, anemia (hematocrit 22%), thrombocytopenia (platelets 17,000/mm^3), and left upper quadrant abdominal fullness. He denies fevers, chills, night sweats, or recent travel outside the United States. He says he has had a heart murmur that his doctor told him was "common and nothing to worry about" for many years. He is a retired wine industry executive and currently consumes 2–3 glasses of wine daily. Physical examination reveals that he is afebrile, pale, and in no distress. His abdominal examination is remarkable for left upper quadrant fullness (Figs. 68.1 and 68.2). A rectal examination reveals brown stool in the rectal vault that is guaiac negative.

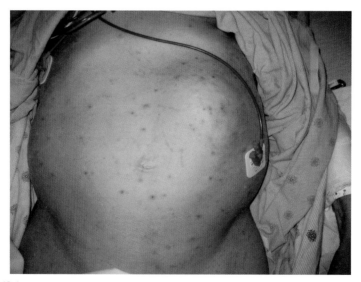

Figure 68.1

Hospital Images: A Clinical Atlas, First Edition. Edited by Paul B. Aronowitz.
© 2012 Wiley-Blackwell. Published 2012 by John Wiley & Sons, Inc.

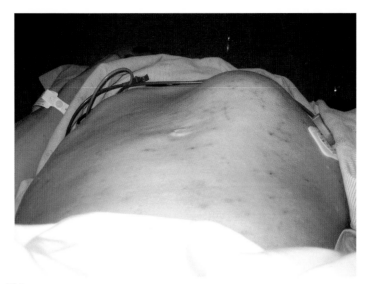

Figure 68.2

Question

Of the following, which is the *most likely* cause of this patient's left upper quadrant fullness?

  A. Malaria
  B. Syphilis
  C. Myelofibrosis
  D. Cirrhosis secondary to chronic alcohol abuse

Answer: B

Although any of these diseases can cause splenomegaly or even massive splenomegaly, hematologic disorders are the most common etiologies of massive splenomegaly in hospitalized patients in the United States. Massive splenomegaly is defined as a spleen 15 centimeters or more below the left costal margin by physical examination or 18 centimeters or greater in length by radiologic study. In one large retrospective study of splenomegaly in hospitalized patients over a 49-year period at a large university medical center, the two most common hematologic disorders causing massive splenomegaly were chronic myelogenous leukemia (CML) and myelofibrosis.

This patient's history is not consistent with infection since he denies fever, chills, and night sweats. He also denies recent travel, making malaria unlikely. While advanced liver disease with portal hypertension can cause massive splenomegaly, this patient's anemia and degree of thrombocytopenia are better explained by a hematologic disorder. Though he does not have signs of infection, syphilis can cause massive splenomegaly and should be considered in the differential diagnosis.

Myelofibrosis is a chronic myeloproliferative disorder characterized by overproduction of megakaryocytes and bone marrow stromal cells. It is characterized by hepatosplenomegaly, normocytic, normochromic anemia, and bone marrow fibrosis. Hepatosplenomegaly results from extramedullary hematopoiesis. Massive splenomegaly can be managed with splenic radiation or splenectomy, but this can result in cytopenias due to the loss of extramedullary hematopoiesis.

O'REILLY RA. Splenomegaly in 2,505 patients at a large university medical center from 1913 to 1995. *West J Med* 1998;169:78–87.

Case 69

A 47-year-old man from North Carolina presents to the Emergency Department with several days of fever, malaise, sore throat, and a maculopapular rash on the palms of his hands (Fig. 69.1) and the soles of his feet (Fig. 69.2). He reports having had sex with men but denies outdoor activities such as hiking, camping, or gardening. He does not recall being bitten by ticks, mosquitoes, or other insects and does not own any pets.

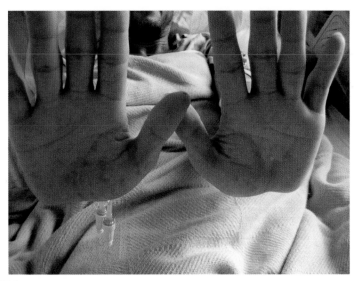

Figure 69.1

Hospital Images: A Clinical Atlas, First Edition. Edited by Paul B. Aronowitz.
© 2012 Wiley-Blackwell. Published 2012 by John Wiley & Sons, Inc.

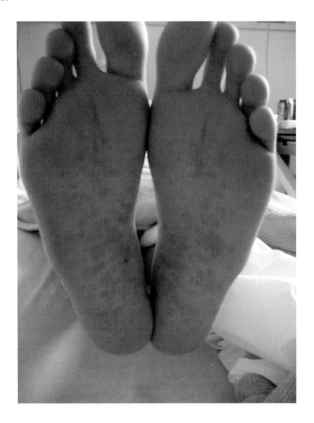

Figure 69.2

Question

What would be the best subsequent step in this patient's management?

    A. Order Rocky Mountain spotted fever serologies and administer intravenous doxycycline.

    B. Culture the lesions on his hands and feet and order a human immunodeficiency virus (HIV) test.

    C. Send blood and throat cultures, order an HIV test, and hold antibiotics pending results.

    D. Send rapid plasma reagin (RPR) and HIV tests and administer penicillin.

Answer: D

This patient's palm and sole maculopapular rash is classic for secondary syphilis. His RPR test was positive at a titre of 1:256 and he was found to be HIV positive. While Rocky Mountain spotted fever should also be considered, there was no history of tick exposure in endemic areas, which are the south central and southeast regions of the United States. The rash of Rocky Mountain spotted fever begins with blanching erythematous macules *around* the wrist and ankles that spreads centripetally, eventually becoming petechial. Of note, the mortality in Rocky Mountain spotted fever rises from 6% in patients in whom treatment is started in the first 5 days of illness to over 20% when treatment is begun after day 5.

Although it is indicated to send an HIV test, culturing the hand and foot lesions would not be practical.

Until the AIDS epidemic, syphilis was rapidly declining in the United States. Concurrent HIV infection should be considered in any patient presenting with syphilis and an HIV test offered. Of patients with secondary syphilis 60–80% develop a rash, which is usually maculopapular, on the palms and soles but it can also occur on the trunk, arms, and legs. Any HIV-positive patient presenting with secondary syphilis and neurologic symptoms should undergo lumbar puncture to search for neurosyphilis. Whether to perform a lumbar puncture in HIV patients without neurologic symptoms is somewhat controversial. Recent studies indicate that in HIV-positive patients without neurologic symptoms who have a CD4 count less than 350 cells per milliliter and/or RPR ≥ 1:32 a lumbar puncture looking for asymptomatic neurosyphilis should strongly be considered.

Secondary syphilis can be treated with one dose of intramuscular penicillin weekly for 3 weeks. If there is neurologic involvement, 2 weeks of intravenous penicillin should be administered.

GHANEM KG, et al. Lumbar puncture in HIV-infected patients with syphilis and no neurologic symptoms. *Clin Infect Dis* 2009;48:816–821.

SINGH AE, ROMANOWSKI B. Syphilis: review with emphasis on clinical, epidemiologic and some biologic features. *Clin Microbiol Rev* 1999:12(2):187–209.

ZETOLA NM, et al. Syphilis in the United States: an update for clinicians with an emphasis on HIV coinfection. *Mayo Clin Proc* 2007;82(9):1091–1102.

Case 70

Image contributed by Jie Yang
Written by Andrea Ling

A 52-year-old male with past medical history of ulcerative colitis is admitted to the hospital after presenting to the Emergency Department with a 3-day history of fever and symmetrical, slightly painful, erythematous papules located on his face, neck, back (Fig. 70.1), and upper extremities (Fig. 70.2). He reports a flu-like illness that resolved more than a week ago.

Physical examination reveals a fever of 39.0°C but his other vital signs are normal. Laboratory studies reveal an elevated white blood cell count of 18,000 cells per microliter with 70% neutrophils. The patient is admitted to the hospital and started on empiric antibiotics by your team. His skin lesions worsen and his fever persists despite the antibiotics.

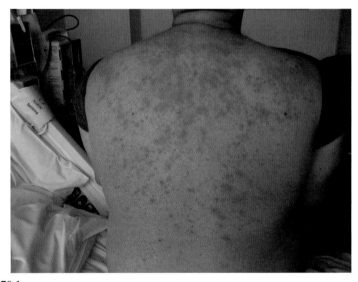

Figure 70.1

Hospital Images: A Clinical Atlas, First Edition. Edited by Paul B. Aronowitz.
© 2012 Wiley-Blackwell. Published 2012 by John Wiley & Sons, Inc.

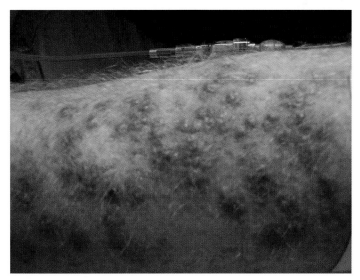

Figure 70.2

Question

Which of the following is this patient's skin disorder *least* likely to be associated with?

   A. Acute myelogenous leukemia
   B. Poison ivy exposure
   C. Nonsteroidal anti-inflammatory drugs (NSAIDs)
   D. A recent viral upper respiratory infection
   E. Inflammatory bowel disease

Answer: B

Sweet's syndrome, also known as acute febrile dermatosis, was described in 1964 by Robert Sweet. It is predominantly seen in women with a mean age of 52 years. Sweet's syndrome is associated with many underlying disorders, which include inflammatory bowel disease, upper respiratory infections (especially streptococcus), and autoimmune disorders such as rheumatoid arthritis and systemic lupus erythematosus. Drugs have also been implicated, with granulocyte colony-stimulating factor (GCSF) being the most commonly reported cause. NSAIDs, antibiotics, and hydralazine can also cause Sweet's syndrome. Hematologic disorders, especially acute myelogenous leukemia, are the etiology in 20–30% of cases of Sweet's syndrome.

Clinically the rash is usually symmetrical, well demarcated, with cutaneous eruptions of erythematous, painful papules and plaques. The lesions can occur anywhere on the body but are most often seen the on face, neck, and upper extremities. Patients may have systemic symptoms such as fever (40–80%), malaise (33%), and conjunctivitis or iridocyclitis (40%).

Laboratory findings are usually nonspecific but may include an elevated erythrocyte sedimentation rate and leukocytosis with a neutrophil predominance.

A skin biopsy is necessary to make the diagnosis. Histologic features include a dense bandlike infiltrate of neutrophils involving mostly the superficial dermis. Standard therapy is oral prednisone with a taper over 2–6 weeks. Response is usually brisk, with fever and leukocytosis resolving in 3 days and skin lesions clearing within 3–9 days. Recurrence is common and may require brief reinstitution of oral steroids. Alternative therapies include potassium iodide and colchicine.

CALLEN J. Neutrophilic dermatoses. *Dermatol Clin* 2002;20:409–419.
FAZILI T. Sweet's syndrome. *Am J Med* 2010;123:694–696.
GUHL G. Subcutaneous Sweet syndrome. *Dermatol Clin* 2008;26:541–551.

Case 71

Image contributed by Andrew Cummins

You are co-managing an 82-year-old man with the neurosurgery service. The patient had evacuation of a right-sided subdural hematoma 1 day ago and was doing well until earlier this morning. You are contacted urgently by the patient's nurse because the patient is unresponsive with decorticate posturing. The neurosurgeon ordered a stat head computerized tomographic (CT) scan (Fig. 71.1) earlier in the morning because the patient seemed "sleepy" and less responsive than on the prior evening. At the time of your examination, you note that there is a Penrose drain exiting the cranium at the site of the previous day's surgery. The patient's right pupil is dilated and unreactive. You contact the neurosurgeon to come and see the patient but he is "stuck in a traffic jam" on his way back to the hospital. The patient's morning laboratory studies are normal except for a serum sodium of 130 mmol/liter, decreased from 138 on the day of surgery.

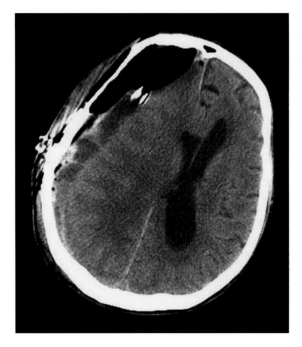

Figure 71.1

Hospital Images: A Clinical Atlas, First Edition. Edited by Paul B. Aronowitz.
© 2012 Wiley-Blackwell. Published 2012 by John Wiley & Sons, Inc.

Question 1

This patient's condition is most consistent with which of the following:

    A. An anaerobic intracranial infection secondary to the surgical procedure

    B. Tension pneumocephalus

    C. Postoperative re-expansion of the subdural hematoma

    D. Hyponatremia due to syndrome of inappropriate antidiuretic hormone (SIADH) from neurosurgery

Question 2

What is the most appropriate subsequent step in this patient's care?

    A. Begin broad-spectrum antibiotics, including metronidazole for anaerobic organism coverage.

    B. If another neurosurgeon cannot be emergently located, consult the primary neurosurgeon by cell phone, access the drain using a 20-gauge needle and syringe, and aspirate.

    C. Begin intravenous 3% saline at a rate of 0.5 mEq per hour.

    D. Contact the patient's family and inform them that the patient will probably not survive the rest of the day.

Answer 1: B

This patient has a large amount of air in his cranium, otherwise known as pneumocephalus (Fig. 71.2, small arrow). The most common cause of pneumocephalus is cranial surgery, but it can also be caused by anaerobic cerebral infections, trauma, tumors, and, rarely, air travel or frequent valsalva maneuvers. This patient's sudden, life-threatening decline in level of conciousness is not simply due to residual air in his cranium. He has a rare complication known as tension pneumocephalus—air is accumulating in the intracranial space without the ability to exit. His CT scan also reveals severe compression of the ventricle with midline shift (Fig. 71.2) and he is clinically showing signs of cerebral herniation.

Although infection should be considered in the differential diagnosis, he is only 1 day postsurgery, making infection much less likely. Re-expansion of the subdural hematoma should also be considered (and was the leading consideration when the neurosurgeon ordered the CT scan earlier in the morning), but the CT scan shows the accumulation of air, not blood. Finally, while this patient's low serum sodium may very well be secondary to neurosurgery or the subdural hematoma, a drop in sodium concentration from 138 to 130 mmol/L is unlikely to explain the precipitous decline in his mental status.

Answer 2: B

Since the neurosurgeon was not available in person, the intern and medical resident caring for this patient consulted with the neurosurgeon by phone. The intern prepared the drain with Betadine and then aspirated 100 cc of serosanguinous material and air present in the intracranial space. The patient markedly improved and, several days later, was transferred to a skilled nursing facility for continued physical and occupational therapy.

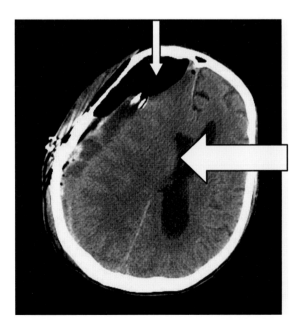

Figure 71.2

CUMMINS A. Tension pneumocephalus is a complication of subdural hematoma evacuation. *J Hosp Med* 2009;4(5):E4.

ISHIWATA Y, et al. Subdural tension pneumocephalus following surgery for chronic subdural hematoma. *J Neurosurg* 1988;68:58–61.

LUO CB, et al. Pneumocephalus secondary to septic thrombosis of the superior sagittal sinus: report of a case. *J Formos Med Assoc* 2001;100(2):142–144.

Case 72

Written by David Jacobson
Image contributed by Kristi Lethert

A 77-year-old woman is admitted from the Emergency Department (ED) with complaints of 2 weeks of headache, neck and scalp pain, and jaw claudication. Physical examination reveals a temperature of 38°C. Her scalp and forehead are not tender and her neurologic examination is normal. You are concerned about the possibility of giant cell arteritis (GCA).

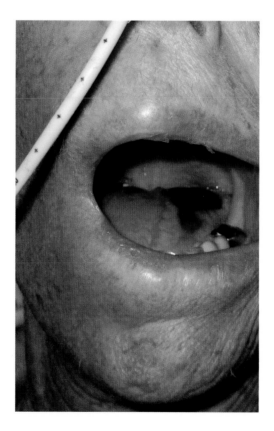

Figure 72.1.

Hospital Images: A Clinical Atlas, First Edition. Edited by Paul B. Aronowitz.
© 2012 Wiley-Blackwell. Published 2012 by John Wiley & Sons, Inc.

Question 1

Regarding giant cell arteritis, which of the following statements is correct?

A. A normal erythrocyte sedimentation rate (ESR) rules out the disease.

B. It is most common in African Americans.

C. The peak incidence occurs between 30 and 50 years of age.

D. Headache is the most sensitive symptom at the time of diagnosis.

The patient's ESR is 68 mm/h and the decision is made to begin steroids.

Question 2

Which of the following statements regarding initial treatment of this disease is correct?

A. Prompt initiation of methylprednisolone usually reverses any visual impairment present at the time of diagnosis.

B. For patients without ocular involvement, a typical starting dose of 10–20 mg of methylprednisolone may be therapeutic and diagnostic.

C. It is preferable to withhold steroids until a temporal artery biopsy can be performed to avoid a false negative result.

D. High-dose steroid therapy with 1000 mg of methylprednisolone for 3 days is recommended for the initial treatment of patients with visual loss.

On hospital day 3 the patient develops unilateral tongue pain (Fig. 72.1).

Question 3

Which of the following statements regarding this disease is *not* correct?

A. Intracranial arteries are more commonly affected than extracranial arteries.

B. Tongue necrosis is a rare complication, resulting from inflammation and thrombosis of the lingual artery.

C. Subclavian artery involvement can result in limb claudication and ischemia.

D. Visual loss is most commonly caused by optic nerve ischemia due to arteritis of the ophthalmic arteries.

The diagnosis of giant cell arteritis is confirmed by temporal artery biopsy revealing granulomatous inflammation with multinucleated giant cells and endovascular thrombus formation. The patient requires local debridement of necrotic tongue tissue and has a slow recovery.

Question 4

Which of the following statements regarding the long-term prognosis and treatment of giant cell arteritis is correct?

A. Few patients with giant cell arteritis exhibit symptoms of polymyalgia rheumatica.

B. Thoracic artery aneurysm is a potential late complication of giant cell arteritis.

C. In most patients, steroid treatment for 6 months or less is usually adequate to induce disease remission.

D. An elevated ESR during follow-up should prompt an increase in corticosteroid dose.

Answer 1: D

Headache is the most sensitive symptom in patients presenting with GCA. Although the majority of patients with GCA have an elevated sedimentation rate, depending upon the case series, anywhere from 0.4% to 22.5% of patients may have a normal ESR. Giant cell arteritis is most common in patients of Scandinavian descent—not African Americans. The peak incidence is in patients age 75–85 and GCA rarely, if ever, occurs in patients less than 50 years of age.

Answer 2: D

High-dose steroid administration with 1000 mg of methylprednisolone for 3 days is recommended for the initial treatment of patients with visual loss. However, visual impairment present at diagnosis rarely improves after initiation of steroids. In polymyalgia rheumatica—not giant cell arteritis—a lower starting dose of 10–20 mg of methylprednisolone is appropriate and may aid in diagnosis. Patients with GCA without ocular involvement typically respond to a daily dose of 40–60 mg of methylprednisolone. Temporal artery biopsy has a high sensitivity if performed within 2 weeks of initiating steroid treatment.

Answer 3: A

Giant cell arteritis affects the extracranial branches of the aorta more frequently than intracranial branches. Tongue necrosis is a well-recognized, though rare, complication of GCA and usually requires debridement. Though thrombosis of the lingual artery is the most common cause of tongue necrosis, other causes of tongue necrosis include syphilis, cancer, and Hodgkin's disease. Limb ischemia and visual loss are both potential complications of GCA. Visual loss is caused by optic nerve ischemia due to arteritis of the ophthalmic artery.

Answer 4: B

Thoracic artery aneurysm is 17 times as likely in patients with GCA as in those without; 40–60% of patients with GCA have symptoms of polymyalgia rheumatica, which can occur before, at the same time as, or after the diagnosis of GCA. Prolonged steroid treatment of 1–2 years' duration is commonly required to treat GCA. The steroid dose should be increased or tapered according to patient symptoms and not by ESR.

GONZALEZ-GAY MA, et al. Giant cell arteritis: laboratory tests at the time of diagnosis in a series of 240 patients. *Medicine* 2005;84:277–290.

SALVARANI C, et al. Polymyalgia rheumatica and giant cell arteritis. *N Engl J Med* 2002;347:261–271.

WEYAND CM, GORONZY JJ. Medium and large-vessel vasculitis. *N Engl J Med* 2003;349:160–169.

Case 73

Image contributed by Vanessa London

An 88-year-old woman with a past medical history of dementia and hypertension is admitted to your service for urosepsis. She had previously smoked cigarettes for 60 years but has not smoked since admission to a nursing home 5 years ago. After assessing the patient and entering admitting orders, the medical intern expresses concern that the patient may have oral cancer. She would like to consult an oral or ear, nose, and throat surgeon to obtain a biopsy.

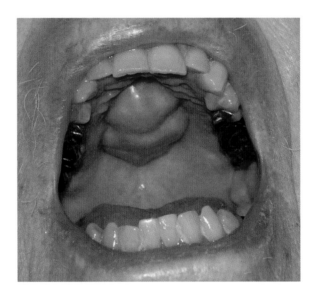

Figure 73.1

Hospital Images: A Clinical Atlas, First Edition. Edited by Paul B. Aronowitz.
© 2012 Wiley-Blackwell. Published 2012 by John Wiley & Sons, Inc.

Question

After examining the patient's oral cavity (Fig. 73.1), what would you tell the intern?

    A. This is most likely squamous cell carcinoma, based upon the location and the patient's history of tobacco use.

    B. This is a pyogenic granuloma.

    C. This is erythroplakia and should be excised since it is a premalignant condition.

    D. This is a congenital anomaly that does not require biopsy or further treatment.

Answer: D

This is a common, benign congenital anomaly that arises from the cortical plate. When located midline in the hard palate this is called torus palatinus and occurs in approximately 25–30% of the population. When located along the lingual aspect of the mandible it is called a torus mandibularis and occurs in 7–10% of the population.

Torus palatinus is twice as common in women as in men and is often not noted until middle age. Surgical consultation would not be indicated in this case unless the torus was interfering with function or with denture fitting (not an issue in this patient since she does not wear dentures) or is subject to refractory surface ulceration from trauma. This patient had a mild speech impediment due to her torus and, despite her dementia, was able to recall that the lesion had been present for many years.

In the United States, oral cancers and oropharyngeal cancers are the ninth most common cancer and account for approximately 3% of malignancies. While this patient is at risk of cancers related to her age and past history of tobacco use, the lesion in this patient's mouth is smooth, symmetric, and otherwise benign appearing.

A pyogenic granuloma is a rapidly growing lesion that occurs in response to irritation. It is usually erythematous, painless, smooth, and bleeds easily. Pyogenic granulomas usually occur on the gingiva but can occasionally occur on the lips, tongue, or buccal mucosa.

Oral leukoplakia is a premalignant condition that appears as a white patch or plaque that cannot be characterized as being due to any other disease. Erythroplakia are analogous red lesions and are more likely than leuoplakia to exhibit dysplasia or carcinoma upon microscopic examination. These lesions tend to occur on the tongue and not midline on the palate.

Gonsalves WC, Chi AC, Neville BW. Common oral lesions: part II. Masses and neoplasia. *Am Fam Phys* 2007;75(4):509–512.

Tran KT, Shannon M. Torus palatinus. *N Engl J Med* 2007;356(17):1759.

Case 74

Written by Susanna Tan
Images contributed by Tom Baudendistel

A 20-year-old woman with a recent history of abscess of the left thigh incised and drained several days prior to admission is admitted to the hospital with a fever of 39.5°C, hypotension, diffuse red rash over her trunk, neck, and arms, and acute kidney failure. She has a healing abscess at her posterior thigh that has a residual 2 × 3-cm area of fluctuance. Over the next 48 hours she is intubated for respiratory failure secondary to adult respiratory distress syndrome (ARDS). On hospital day 7, she develops diffuse desquamation of the skin on her hands (Figs. 74.1 and 74.2), face (Fig. 74.3), arms, and trunk.

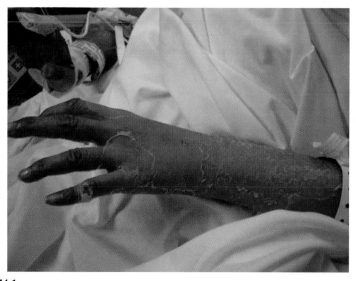

Figure 74.1

Hospital Images: A Clinical Atlas, First Edition. Edited by Paul B. Aronowitz.
© 2012 Wiley-Blackwell. Published 2012 by John Wiley & Sons, Inc.

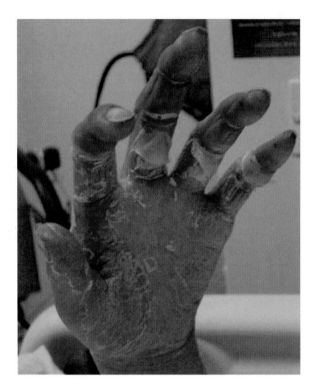

Figure 74.2

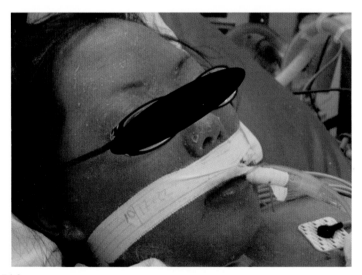

Figure 74.3

Question 1

Which of the following is *least* likely to be helpful in the treatment of this disorder?

A. Antibiotic coverage for *Clostridium perfringens* and *Bacteroides fragilis*

B. "Early goal-directed therapy"

C. Early surgical exploration and debridement of her thigh abscess

D. Administration of intravenous immunoglobulins (IVIG)

Question 2

Which patient population is most at risk of developing this disorder?

A. Menstruating women using superabsorbent tampons

B. Women using barrier contraceptive devices

C. Patients with postoperative wound infections

D. All the above

Answer 1: A

Toxic shock syndrome (TSS) is a toxin-mediated, acute, life-threatening illness, characterized by high fever, rash, hypotension, and, frequently, multiorgan failure. Desquamation tends to occur 1–2 weeks after the onset of illness. TSS is typically precipitated by exotoxins released from *Staphylococcus aureus* or group A *Streptococcus*. The toxin serves as a superantigen, with the ability to trigger excessive T-cell activation with consequent downstream activation of other cell types along with cytokine release. Treatment for toxic shock involves immediate early goal-directed therapy, antibiotic coverage against *Staphylococcus* and *Streptococcus* species, and source control with early debridement of infected wounds. IVIG has been found to have significant neutralizing activity against the TSS exotoxin.

Answer 2: D

Fifty percent of cases of toxic shock syndrome are not associated with menstruation and use of superabsorbent tampons. While the incidence of nonmenstrual TSS has remained relatively constant, the incidence of menstrual TSS has decreased, possibly due to increased awareness. Nonmenstrual cases of TSS have been associated with the use of barrier contraceptives, surgical and postpartum wound infections, cutaneous infections (as in this case), and burns.

ANDREWS MM, et al. Recurrent nonmenstrual toxic shock syndrome: clinical manifestations, diagnosis, and treatment. *Clin Infect Dis* 2001;32(10):1470–1479.

LAPPIN E, FERGUSON AJ. Gram-positive toxic shock syndromes. *Lancet Infect Dis* 2009;9(5):281–290.

YANAGISAWA C, et al. Neutralization of staphylococcal exotoxins in vitro by human-origin intravenous immunoglobulin. *J Infect Chemother* 2007;13(6):368–372.

Case 75

Image contributed by Albert Lu
Written by Aaron Falk

A 58-year-old man with a history of type II diabetes mellitus presents to the Emergency Department (ED) in November with fever and dyspnea. He reports that he developed severe myalgias 4 days prior to admission and that his symptoms rapidly progressed to include generalized malaise, fever, and nausea. Over the prior 24 hours he developed a nonproductive cough and worsening shortness of breath.

The patient reports that several of his co-workers have been absent from work because of the "flu." Physical examination reveals an ill-appearing man in mild respiratory distress with a temperature of 39.0°C, blood pressure 128/82 mmHg, pulse 101, respiratory rate 24, and oxygen saturation of 92% on room air. Respiratory examination reveals bilateral, diffuse crackles but he is without jugular venous distention or peripheral edema. A rapid antigen influenza test is ordered and returns positive. There are two other patients in the ED with positive influenza tests. His admission chest radiograph is shown in Figure 75.1.

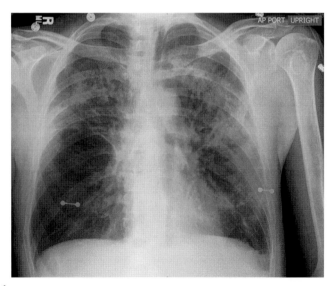

Figure 75.1

Hospital Images: A Clinical Atlas, First Edition. Edited by Paul B. Aronowitz.
© 2012 Wiley-Blackwell. Published 2012 by John Wiley & Sons, Inc.

Question 1

Which medication should be administered to this patient as the best subsequent step in his management?

A. Amantadine

B. Oseltamivir

C. Ceftriaxone and azithromycin

D. Furosemide

Question 2

Which statement correctly describes commercially available rapid antigen tests for influenza?

A. A positive test in this patient likely represents a true positive.

B. Tests are highly sensitive for influenza.

C. A diagnostic test is not needed given this patient's "classic" presentation.

D. A positive test should be confirmed with culture before starting treatment.

Answer 1: B

This patient has primary influenza pneumonia. Patients typically present with dyspnea and cough in addition to the "classic symptoms" of influenza, which include fever and myalgias. Occasionally primary influenza pneumonia is so severe that patients present with cyanosis. The radiologic appearance of primary influenza pneumonia is widely variable and can range from a normal-appearing chest radiograph to lobar infiltrates that mimic bacterial pneumonia. This patient's chest radiograph shows bilateral infiltrates in a "batwing" configuration suggesting widespread involvement. Secondary bacterial pneumonia is a common pulmonary complication of influenza and may account for up to 25% of influenza-related deaths. In contrast to this patient, who developed pneumonia almost immediately after his initial influenza infection, a patient with secondary bacterial pneumonia will typically have a transient improvement prior to the onset of pulmonary symptoms.

Oseltamivir, a neuraminidase inhibitor, is the appropriate treatment for acute influenza. Oseltamivir is active against both influenza A and influenza B, whereas amantadine is active only against influenza A and is not currently recommended for empiric treatment of influenza infection. Ceftriaxone and azithromycin would be appropriate treatment for bacterial community-acquired pneumonia; however, they are not active against the influenza virus. There is no evidence that this patient is in heart failure and furosemide would not be an appropriate treatment. Additionally, there is not adequate evidence to suggest that diuresis improves outcomes in patients with influenza pneumonia.

Answer 2: A

As with other diagnostic tests, it is important to consider pre-test probability when interpreting laboratory results. Rapid antigen testing has a sensitivity of only 40–60%, so testing patients with a low pre-test probability of influenza infection may not be useful. Since this patient reports having been exposed to others with influenza and has a history and examination consistent with influenza pneumonia, the pre-test probability of his having influenza is quite high. In this setting a positive rapid antigen test very likely represents a true positive. Most clinicians would recommend a diagnostic test in this patient because of his severity of illness and the need to exclude other diagnoses. In patients with a typical presentation of influenza during an outbreak and less-severe illness, treatment without diagnostic testing is acceptable. It would not be appropriate to delay treatment to wait for culture results—antiviral therapy should be started immediately.

CALL SA, et al. Does this patient have influenza? *JAMA* 2005;293(8):987–997.

HARPER SA, et al. Seasonal influenza in adults and children—diagnosis, treatment, chemoprophylaxis, and institutional outbreak management: clinical practice guidelines of the Infectious Diseases Society of America. *Clin Infect Dis* 2009;48(8):1003–1032.

Case 76

Written by Aaron Falk

An 85-year-old man with a history of chronic atrial fibrillation who takes warfarin for stroke prophylaxis is admitted to the hospital for 1 day of abdominal pain that began in the left upper quadrant. The intensity of the pain progressed and on presentation to the Emergency Department he describes severe pain in a bandlike distribution across the abdomen in the upper quadrants. He denies fever or recent trauma. The morning of presentation he had a normal bowel movement. Physical examination reveals stable vital signs. His abdomen is mildly tender without rebound tenderness and his stool is positive for occult blood with guaiac testing. Initial laboratory data includes a white blood cell count of 7.8 g/dL and platelets of 179,000/μL. His international normalized ratio (INR) is 9.1. A computerized tomographic (CT) scan of the abdomen and pelvis shows a 20-cm segment of thickened small bowel in the right pelvis (Fig. 76.1, arrow).

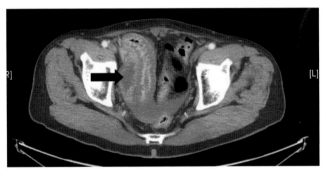

Figure 76.1

Hospital Images: A Clinical Atlas, First Edition. Edited by Paul B. Aronowitz.
© 2012 Wiley-Blackwell. Published 2012 by John Wiley & Sons, Inc.

Question 1

What is the best subsequent step in this patient's management?

   A. Reverse the patient's coagulopathy and observe.
   B. Perform an emergent laparotomy.
   C. Obtain an emergent CT angiogram.
   D. Use capsule endoscopy to evaluate the small bowel.

Question 2

What is the most appropriate treatment in reversing this patient's coagulopathy?

   A. Vitamin K administered via subcutaneous route
   B. Oral vitamin K
   C. Oral vitamin K and 2 units of fresh frozen plasma (FFP)
   D. Intravenous vitamin K and 2 units of FFP

Answer 1: A

This patient has a spontaneous intramural hematoma of the small bowel secondary to supra-therapeutic anticoagulation. Small bowel hematomas are a common complication of trauma to the abdomen, but spontaneous occurrence has been reported in association with a coagu-lopathic state. The most common underlying cause of spontaneous small bowel hematoma is warfarin toxicity, but it has also been reported with conditions such as leukemia. Presenting symptoms include pain and gastrointestinal bleeding. There are case reports of extensive hematomas leading to small bowel obstruction. The prognosis is favorable when the coagu-lopathy can be reversed, thus avoiding surgical exploration.

Bowel ischemia should be considered in any patient with abdominal pain, atrial fibrilla-tion, and thickened bowel wall, but this patient's supratherapeutic INR makes this diagnosis much less likely. Capsule endoscopy is not needed in this case and would most likely be contraindicated given the extensive abnormality in the small bowel and the increased likeli-hood of capsule retention.

Answer 2: C

This patient is actively bleeding and it would be appropriate to urgently correct his coagu-lopathy. Vitamin K can be used to reverse the effects of warfarin toxicity but its effects will take several hours. Immediate correction of the coagulopathy can be achieved with fresh frozen plasma. Whenever possible, vitamin K should be given by mouth. Subcutaneous injec-tions of vitamin K are unreliably absorbed, and intravenous administration carries the risk of anaphylaxis.

ABBAS MA, et al. Spontaneous intramural small-bowel hematoma: clinical presentation and long-term outcome. *Arch Surg* 2002;137:306–310.

LUBETSKY A, et al. Comparison of oral vs intravenous phytonadione (vitamin K1) in patients with exces-sive anticoagulation: a prospective randomized controlled study. *Arch Intern Med* 2003;163(20): 2469–2473.

Index

Hospital Images: A Clinical Atlas, First Edition. Edited by Paul B. Aronowitz.
© 2012 Wiley-Blackwell. Published 2012 by John Wiley & Sons, Inc.